D0197750

THE COMPLETE GUIDE TO
SPORTS INJURIES

WITHDRAWN

EFC Library

757365

THE COMPLETE GUIDE TO
SPORTS INJURIES

Christopher M. Norris

A & C Black • London

EPPING FOREST COLLEGE LIBRARY
BORDERS LANE, LOUGHTON
ESSEX IG10 3SA
Tel: 020 8508 8311

757365

Note

Whilst every effort has been made to ensure that the content of this book is as technically accurate and as sound as possible, neither the author nor the publishers can accept responsibility for any injury or loss sustained as a result of the use of this material.

Published by A&C Black Publishers Ltd, an imprint of
Bloomsbury Publishing Plc
36 Soho Square, London W1D 3QY
www.acblack.com

Copyright © 2011 Christopher M. Norris

ISBN 978 1 4081 3077 3

All rights reserved. No part of this publication may be reproduced in any form or by any means – graphic, electronic or mechanical, including photocopying, recording, taping or information storage and retrieval systems – without the prior permission in writing of the publishers.

Christopher M. Norris has asserted his rights under the Copyright, Design and Patents Act, 1988, to be identified as the author of this work.

A CIP catalogue record for this book is available from the British Library.

Acknowledgements

Inside photographs © Laura Scott-Burns with the exception of the following:
© Grant Pritchard pp 55 (top), 62 (bottom), 67, 89, 102, 112, 120, 130, 132; © Pro-Tech Athletics pp 11, 61, 78; © Physique pp 11 (left), 14, 15; ©Physiosupplies p 12; © Thumper Massage Inc. p 15 (top) ThumperMini Pro2 is a registered trademark of Thumper Massager Inc.; Swede-O, Inc. p 190, © Shutterstock p 20.

Illustrations

All illustrations courtesy of David Gardner with the exception of the following:
© Jeff Edwards pp 31, 33, 117, 127, 128

Cover photograph © Getty Images

Cover and text designed by James Watson

This book is produced using paper that is made from wood grown in managed, sustainable forests. It is natural, renewable and recyclable. The logging and manufacturing processes conform to the environmental regulations of the country of origin.

Typeset in 10.75pt Adobe Caslon on 14pt by Saxon Graphics Ltd, Derby

Printed and bound in China by C & C Offset Printing

CONTENTS

PREFACE

The Complete Guide to Sports Injuries provides a link between the work of a clinician and that of a fitness professional. Written for the non-specialist it aims to strike a balance between the theory base of science on the one hand, and the practical elements of injury management on the other. The book begins with a description of *how tissues heal* in chapter 1 because an understanding of these mechanisms underpins all successful treatment. We then look at *your treatment toolbox* – it may come as some surprise that you do not need complex or expensive equipment to effectively manage sports injuries. There is a focus on hands-on techniques; in particular and we look at massage, taping, hot and cold. Chapter 3 examines *structuring rehabilitation* because exercise therapy is the linchpin of sports injury management right through the whole of the healing process. Whether it be managing a sprain or tear or aiming to return to sport after surgery, exercise therapy is the single most important component of any treatment programme. The book is packed full of photographs and diagrams to aid both understanding and technique, and aims to be an essential introduction for all those involved in the care of injured sports personnel. It is important to note that this book is not designed to replace a trip to the physiotherapist or GP, but to help you become one of the team who manages injuries successfully.

Christopher M. Norris, 2011

HOW TISSUES HEAL

1

When you are managing sports injuries, it is essential to understand the process that tissues go through as they heal so that you can work with your body's healing rather than against it. As healing progresses, treatment will change, so knowledge of the healing timescale is vital. The changes occurring within the healing tissues and the parallel changes which you cause with treatment must closely match if you are to achieve a satisfactory return to sport.

INJURY AND INFLAMMATION

The moment you sustain a sports injury your tissues begin to heal. The process is continuous right up until the point where you have full function of your body part and can return to sport. For convenience the healing process can be divided into four interrelated phases (*see* fig 1.1). Let's begin by looking at the first phase, injury.

INJURY

When soft tissue, such as muscle or ligaments, is damaged some of the local blood capillaries which run through it are disrupted, releasing fresh blood into the area. This has two important effects. First, as you will see later, the tissue disruption instigates chemical messages which begin the healing process. Second, because the blood vessels

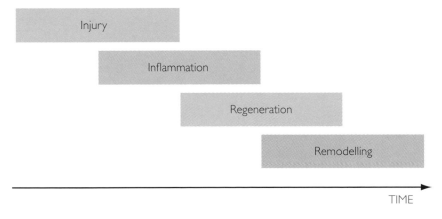

Figure 1.1 Phases of healing

are damaged, fresh blood can no longer flow into the local tissues. Starved of new blood, which should bring with it oxygen and tissue nutrients, the tissues begin to die. Think of this like watering your garden: if you cut the hosepipe no water gets to the flowers and they dry up and die. The same is true here, except it is a blood vessel which has been cut and your tissue rather than your flowers which may wither. If you continue to exercise, the metabolic rate or 'tick over' of the tissues remains high and the demand for oxygen is increased. This increased demand speeds up tissue death which is occurring due to the oxygen shortage. Rest is therefore vital to slow the metabolic rate and reduce the oxygen demand. As we will see later there are several other actions you can use to reduce the oxygen demand of your tissues, and this is the best treatment you can offer your body to work with your natural healing processes.

Definition

Metabolic rate is the chemical 'tick over' of the body. It is the amount of oxygen and nutrients that your body requires just to keep going. Exercise increases metabolic rate, while rest reduces it – much like putting your foot on a car accelerator pedal to use more petrol, and taking it off to use less.

Local cell death occurring in the injured tissues releases enzymes which begin the process of digesting and dissolving dead material. The body acts quickly as a natural 'road sweeper' to clean up the area in preparation for new tissue growth. This activity further stimulates the release of important chemicals including *histamine* and *prostaglandin* which act as chemical messengers.

As blood is released by damaged blood vessels, red blood cells are damaged, causing blood clotting to begin. The blood chemical *fibrin* beings to form a meshwork around the injured area, which then develops into a clot. The blood clot is an essential precursor to form a bridge between the ends of the torn tissue, and any movement which disrupts the clot slows the normal healing process. Continuing to exercise in the immediate post-injury phase is therefore detrimental.

Keypoint

Immediately after injury your tissues are disrupted and their blood flow reduced. Starved of new blood, tissue death will occur. Rest is vital to slow this process down.

INFLAMMATION

Inflammation begins 10 minutes after an injury occurs and may last several days depending on the sports first-aid action which is taken. Inflammation gives four outward signs: *heat*, *redness*, *swelling* and *pain* (*see* fig 1.2, page 3).

Heat and *redness* occur due to the increase in local blood flow, that is blood which flows close to the injured area. This increase develops as a result of blood vessels opening. Just as your skin becomes red as you exercise and get hot in the gym, the local skin surrounding an injury reddens. However, this will only be noticeable where the damaged tissues are close to the surface (superficial). When you sprain your ankle, the area feels hot and looks red, but if you damage your back, where the

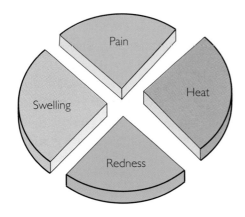

Figure 1.2 Signs of inflammation

damaged tissues lie much deeper, the area may feel hot to you but, to an outside observer, redness is rarely noticeable unless the condition is very severe. Again, the process is brought about by a number of chemicals including *prostaglandin*, and it is on this chemical that anti-inflammatory drugs such as NSAIDs work to calm the process of inflammation.

> **Definition**
>
> An *NSAID* is a non-steroidal anti-inflammatory drug (e.g. ibuprofen) which is used to reduce pain and inflammation, especially of joint and muscle conditions.

The broken blood vessels cause blood flow to slow. The blood cells themselves become sticky, adhering to the vessel walls to form part of the developing blood clot which dams the area to stop further bleeding into the damaged tissues.

Swelling (also called *oedema*) begins as the slow blood movement is unable to keep pace with the fluids being formed by the body. As the damaged tissues release their chemicals, the body tries to dilute the area with watery fluid, which is the basis of swelling. The swelling moves into the lymphatic vessels and should be taken away as part of the normal lymph flow process.

> **Definition**
>
> The *lymphatic system* is a network of fine tubes which exists in additional to the blood vessels. Blood does not directly contact tissues; instead, the blood cells remain in the vessels and a clear fluid called *lymph* seeps out to touch the tissues directly. It is the lymph fluid which runs within the lymphatic system.

Unfortunately, the sheer volume of swelling which often develops after a sports injury means that some fluid will settle and pool around the injured area. Initially, the swelling is a watery fluid, but it contains similar clotting chemicals to blood and, over time, will become firmer and gel-like. If left, over many weeks the gel-like swelling can still harden further. One of our aims should be to restrict the spread of this sticky swelling so that it affects a smaller area. This is one function of elastic supports and taping. Another of our tools can be massage, which aims to remove excess swelling and stave off the problem of the tissue becoming stuck together (consolidated oedema). As you will see in chapter 2, while massage helps the healing process by removing swelling, if used too early or too vigorously it can disrupt the healing process and slow the recovery.

Keypoint

Following injury you must aim to stem the spread of swelling.

Pain is an inevitable consequence of sports injuries and occurs because the chemicals produced at the time of injury irritate the nerve sensors within the tissues. As swelling occurs, the pressure of the developing fluids presses on the sensors and further pain is produced. Pain is created by tiny electrical nervous impulses travelling from the tissue sensors to the brain. This feeling (sensory) mechanism consists of nerves which travel as a *pain pathway*, firstly to the spinal cord. Here, they form a junction (synapse) with a small intermediate nerve (interneuron) which itself connects to a longer fibre travelling to the brain, where the pain is actually felt. Even within the brain, there are several nerve connections (*see* fig 1.3, page 5). At each junction between the nerves, the nervous impulse can be changed. This fact is important both for pain relief and for the development of longer-term (chronic) pain. If another nerve impulse arrives at the nerve junction in the spine, it can cancel out the painful signal. This is what happens when you knock your knee and 'rub it better'. The vigorous rubbing causes an intense sensory stimulus which cancels out the pain at the level of the spinal cord – an effect called *counter-irritation*.

As the nerve impulse travels into the brain, you feel pain (sensory perception). However, the impulse also travels across junctions to other nerves going to different brain areas. Some go to emotional centres, and so intense pain, especially if it occurs over a prolonged period, can cause emotional changes such as fear of movement. Fear of this type is important to consider when a personal trainer gives a client exercise following a severe injury such as a broken leg from a car accident, for example.

Definition

A *counter-irritant effect* is caused when a second intense stimulus cancels out a painful feeling. The effect occurs at the junction between two sensory nerves.

The nerve junctions can also work to our advantage. You can reduce or block pain using treatments such as heat, massage and ice. Impulses produced by the brain as a result of these treatments can flood the body with pain-relieving chemicals and also remove the fear of movement. This type of pain relief is called *descending inhibition* and it is caused by many of the treatment tools you will use in chapter 2. Both descending inhibition and the reduction of fear of movement are known to occur when using exercise. The use of graded exercise programmes with patients suffering from chronic pain, for example, is now at the forefront of pain research.

THE HEALING TIMESCALE

The process of tissue healing can take some time. Minor knocks may resolve in a matter of days, while more major injuries can take many months and sometimes even years to heal completely. The

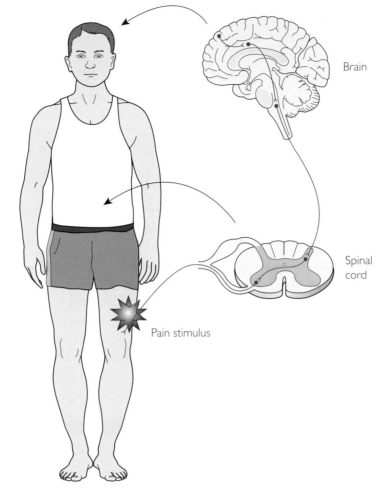

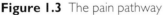

Pain stimulus

Figure 1.3 The pain pathway

key to the healing timescale is the amount of tissue damage you have and how the injury is treated. The process of healing described previously proceeds through three interrelated phases: *acute*, *sub-acute* and *chronic*.

• During the *acute* phase your tissues have been damaged and are reacting to this. It is the stage of *inflammation*. There is local bleeding and

swelling. Your tissues have only begun to heal slowly, and so your aim should be damage limitation – you must not take any action that could stress the damaged tissues and further injure them. It is a sad fact that in some cases there can be more tissue damage induced by trying to run an injury off, or play with painkillers blocking out the pain, than actually occurred at the time of injury. In addition, we have seen that the swelling formed at the time of injury can spread throughout the local area. Limiting this spread is vital because the sticky swelling will clot, and if it travels further there will be more tissue affected. The acute phase of healing typically lasts 48 hours and ceases when the tissues begin to form a healing bridge across the damaged area.

• When the healing tissues start to form and no fresh swelling or bleeding occurs, you have entered the *sub-acute* phase of healing, which may last anything from 14 to 21 days. This is the stage of *regeneration* when tissue regrowth begins. Initially, a soft blood clot forms and a stronger tissue mesh begins to grow around the area. The new healing tissue forms a scar in the same way that the skin heals after a cut. This tissue shrinks and pulls its torn ends together, effectively bridging the tissue gap. The tissue formed at this stage of healing has fibres which are arranged in a haphazard fashion. The finished tissue must have fibres which align in the strongest direction possible (organised) – a topic discussed in the section on scar tissue below.

• The final stage of the healing timescale is the *chronic* phase, which is the stage of *remodelling* lasting from 21 days onwards. Although the term 'chronic' is used here, this phase is an essential stage in which your scar tissue adapts to become more like the original tissue it has replaced. Again, exercise is vital, and if the exercise is too gentle, the tissue will not be stressed sufficiently to adapt fully. The tissue stress must not just be intense, but must closely match that which will be used in sport.

In other words, the stresses imposed on the healed tissue must be *functional*, a topic covered in chapter 3.

The remodelling phase can last for many years, and one of the mistakes which is often made during rehabilitation is to stop too soon. Although your tissue may be relatively pain free when healed by 80%, it is still not fully functional. In other words, when subjected to the severe stress of competitive sport, your tissue may fail. It is vital during this phase that a sportsperson has a graded rehabilitation programme which lasts long enough – at least 3–4 months. Many of us find this odd, saying, 'surely my injury will not last that long'. However, saying this misses an essential phase of healing – that of tissue adaptation. If you join a gym and begin performing a bench press, you should expect to improve the weight you are able to lift over a period of time. The improvement is a result of tissue adaptation, with the chest and arm muscles (pectorals and triceps) getting stronger. You would not just give up in a matter of weeks, but would continue with your programme over months and years. Why? Because you know that the muscles will continue to strengthen providing your training is correct. The same is true of tissue adaptation following injury. If the rehab programme is correct, tissue adaptation will continue for many months.

SCAR TISSUE

We have seen that new tissue is formed as healing progresses. This tissue is a meshwork of fibres formed from fibrous tissue. Fibrous tissue contains two main types of fibre: one which is strong (fibrin) and the other more elastic (elastin). The

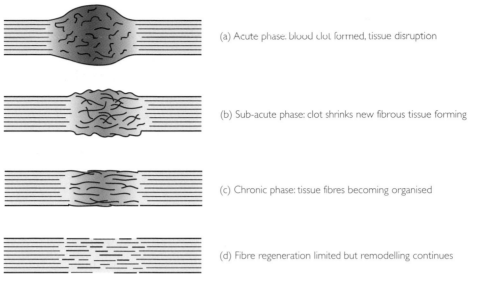

(a) Acute phase: blood clot formed, tissue disruption

(b) Sub-acute phase: clot shrinks new fibrous tissue forming

(c) Chronic phase: tissue fibres becoming organised

(d) Fibre regeneration limited but remodelling continues

Figure 1.4 Phases of tissue healing

amount of each of these fibres is governed by the requirements of the tissue. For example, both the tendons at the ends of muscles and the ligaments which support joints are made of fibrous tissue.

However, ligaments are more stretchy than tendons and so have a greater proportion of elastin fibres than fibrin. As your injury heals, it is vital that your tissue remodels to closely resemble the original tissue format. If it is too loose or too tight, its function will be impaired. The make-up of fibrous tissue changes depending on the stress placed upon it.

We have seen that after injury a blood clot forms (*see* fig 1.4a) and shrinks (*see* fig 1.4b). The healing meshwork of fibrous tissue which begins to form has a haphazard appearance with fibres pointing in various directions (*see* fig 1.4c). The finished tissue must have fibres which align in the strongest direction possible (*see* fig 1.4d) and take on the function of the original tissue.

To change from the haphazard fibre orientation to a more organised mesh, the tissue must be stressed slightly: with too little stress the fibres will not align correctly; with too much, the fibres will break down again. In the sub-acute phase progressive exercise is the key. Here, gentle exercise is chosen which increases in intensity to match the developing strength of the healing tissues.

Keypoint

During healing progressive exercise is vital. Tissues must be stressed to encourage strong fibre development. The stress must match the strength of the newly formed tissue.

7

MUSCLE ADAPTATION TO INJURY AND DISUSE

One of the tissues which is most affected by any injury is muscle. It will become weaker and shrink (waste) due to pain. Muscle wastage occurs through changes in nervous impulses. Normally, even at rest your muscles receive constant nerve impulses to keep them ready for action. This *resting tone*, as it is called, gives your muscle its natural firmness. The tone reduces if the muscle is not used, because fewer nervous impulses get through. The flabby muscle appearance is called *disuse atrophy*.

When a joint swells and is painful, the body tries to protect itself by preventing movement. Now, the muscle tone drops off very quickly (within 24 hours). In this case it is not just a reduction in nervous impulses which normally tell the muscle to stay firm, but an increase in other impulses which deliberately tell the muscle to relax – a condition called *muscular inhibition*. Moving a painful joint will increase these new nervous impulses and intensify the muscular inhibition. Protecting a painful swollen joint from movement is therefore vital and is the job of taping and splinting (*see* chapter 2).

Definition

Disuse atrophy is muscle wasting due to lack of use; *muscle inhibition* is wasting due to nerve impulses created by pain and swelling.

Following injury it is vital that your muscle strength be increased to pre-injury levels. There are a number of considerations here, however.

First, muscle will not strengthen effectively where pain still exists. Strength training produces nerve signals telling a muscle to increase its tone, while pain produces other signals telling the muscle to reduce tone. The result is that the two forms of stimuli cancel each other out and the muscle does not strengthen. Gentle exercise may be used when pain is present to increase the flow of fluids (blood and lymph) around the area, but pain should never increase. Once pain has subsided, gentle exercise may give way to strengthening (*see* chapter 3).

The second consideration when using exercise is the presence of *movement dysfunction*. Here, the quality of a movement will have degraded due to pain. An everyday example of movement dysfunction is a limp. When you get a stone in your shoe, the pressure on the sole of your foot causes you to change the way you walk to avoid the pain. With each step you are in fact practising a new form of walking – literally rehearsing your limp. After some time, if you take the stone out of your shoe, you will still limp because you have now practised the movement dysfunction and it has become a habit. If you decide to use walking as part of a training programme, you will be further reinforcing the movement dysfunction and, although you may walk faster because you have increased your

Keypoint

It is important to correct *movement quality* (how you perform an exercise) before *movement quantity* (how many repetitions of an exercise you can do).

movement quantity, the movement quality is poor. It is therefore vital to undo the limp (correct the movement dysfunction) before you increase the amount of exercise you do. One of the fundamental underpinnings of rehabilitation is to address movement quality before movement quantity.

Terms you should know:

Basal metabolic rate (BMR) – the speed of chemical reactions when the body is at rest.

Consolidated oedema – swelling which has become firm. When pressed, an impression of the fingertip is left behind. Also called *pitting oedema*.

Counter-irritation – relieving pain by introducing a second (intense) sensory stimulus.

Disuse atrophy – muscle wasting due to lack of use.

Fibrin – a blood chemical involved in clotting.

Fibrous tissue – non-contracting general soft tissue.

Inflammation – the first part of the tissue healing process. Inflammation is recognised by heat, redness, swelling and pain.

Histamine – a chemical messenger involved in tissue healing which triggers the inflammatory response.

Interneuron – small connecting nerve lying between two longer nerves.

Lymph – fluid found both between body cells and flowing within lymphatic vessels. Also called *interstitial fluid*.

Metabolic rate – the speed of chemical reactions in the body.

Movement dysfunction – a reduced quality of movement (e.g. limping).

Muscle inhibition – muscle wasting due to nerve impulses resulting from pain and swelling.

NSAID – an acronym for *non-steroidal anti-inflammatory drug*.

Oedema (swelling) – the medical term for swelling: the accumulation of fluid beneath the skin. Called *edema* in America.

Prostaglandin – a chemical messenger involved in tissue healing which causes vasodilation.

Synapse – junction between two nerves.

Vasodilation – expansion or opening of blood vessels to increase blood flow in tissue.

YOUR TREATMENT TOOLBOX

2

We have seen in chapter 1 that one of the major aims of sports first-aid treatment is to limit further tissue damage which occurs as a result of the reduction in blood flow at the time of injury. Remember, tearing of the blood capillaries allows local blood to flood into the area, while at the same time nutrients and oxygen do not reach the tissue cells. Further cell death can occur if the metabolic rate (speed of chemical reactions) of the tissues is increased by exercising. We limit the likelihood of tissue damage using a procedure indicated by the mnemonic *PRICE*.

PRICE

PRICE stands for *Protect, Rest, Ice, Compression* and *Elevation* and is a simple method for planning the initial management of a sports injury.

- To prevent further tissue damage we begin with the word **protect**. This single term helps us remember several important aspects. First, we must rest rather than trying to work an injury off. This may simply require us to, for example, sit on a chair with our foot up on a stool. However, if we are on the field or in a gym, we have to get home and may require crutches or a stick to protect the injured area.

Alternatively, we may use a splint (*see* fig 2.1a, page 11) to prevent unnecessary movement of a limb. Compression may be used from an elastic bandage (such as tubigrip), and rigid taping may be used only where it does not restrict the blood flow to the limb (*see* below).

- **Rest** is important to allow time for the injured tissues to heal. The amount of rest will be dependent on the volume of tissue affected. Large injuries may require total rest to allow the body to recover in the initial hours after injury. This is because a combination of tissue damage and pain can result in shock, causing the blood pressure to reduce and making you feel light-headed and off colour. More minor injuries will only require rest of the body part affected. For example, a person with tennis elbow needs to rest the elbow itself, but also avoid certain shoulder actions which may affect the elbow. However, they can still exercise the legs and abdomen to maintain fitness. As healing progresses, rest is adapted in parallel. Here we use *functional rest* – avoiding only actions which place strain on the tissues that were injured. Take an example of a sprained ankle (*see* chapter 4). The most common injury

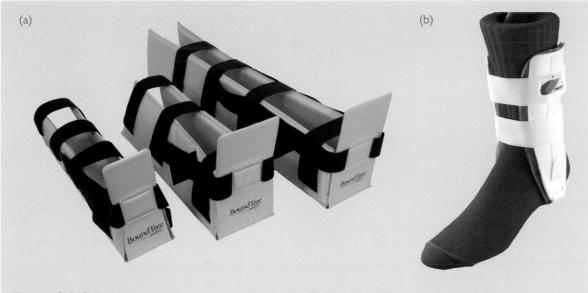

Figure 2.1 Splints to immobilise a joint: (a) rigid splint (Frack splint) (b) ankle immobiliser

is to the ligament on the outside of the joint, and this is stretched when the foot is pointed downwards and inwards (plantar flexion and inversion). As part of functional rest, we can tape the ankle to limit this movement only, but allow other movements to occur freely.

> ### Keypoint
> *Functional rest* avoids using only those actions which place stress on the injured tissues. All other movements may be used freely to maintain fitness.

- **Ice** or cold is used as part of sports first aid to reduce the metabolic demands of the local tissues by placing them in a state of temporary hibernation. As we will discuss later, in the later stages of rehabilitation ice may also be used to increase blood flow and reduce pain. Placing ice directly onto the skin is very dangerous. Because ice from a freezer is actually at a lower temperature than normal ice it may cause a severe ice burn. The outer layers of skin rapidly go white and die, although the numbing effect of the ice fails to alert you that there is a problem. This is particularly dangerous on thinner structures such as the Achilles tendon where blistering may occur. To prevent this problem, use ice wrapped in a moist cloth so that there is a layer of iced water between the ice cubes and the skin. Where ice bags are used (*see* fig 2.2, overleaf), again these should be wrapped in a damp cloth – a tea towel is ideal. The cold pack should be left on for 15 minutes and reapplied every 2 hours throughout the daytime, roughly twice in the morning and three times in the afternoon and evening. Continue this application for the first two days (48 hours) until the acute inflammation has settled.

Keypoint

Apply a moist cold pack for 15 minutes every 2 hours throughout the waking day, for 48 hours following an injury. *Never* put fresh ice from the freezer directly onto unprotected skin – a serious ice burn (blistering and skin death) may occur.

• As fluid accumulates following injury, swelling appears on the body surface. We have seen that the sticky fluid will attach to local tissues and solidify eventually, giving consolidated oedema if left. To prevent the accumulation and spread of this fluid, we use **compression**. One of the simplest ways to supply this is to use commercially available elastic stocking bandage such as tubigrip. This type of bandage provides uniform compression and conforms to the limb – two important requirements. Uniform compression prevents the formation of fluid pockets and conforming to the limb means that pressure is not placed over prominent areas. Taking the example of the ankle above, if excessive pressure is placed over the ankle bones (malleoli), the skin covering the area can chafe and break down. Uniform compression is provided by the bandage stretching more over larger areas of the calf and less around the ankle. In this way a pocket of swelling is less likely to form around the bottom of the outer ankle bone (lateral malleolus), where it tends to congregate through the natural pull of gravity. Sometimes more compression is required, however, and a *compression bandage* is used.

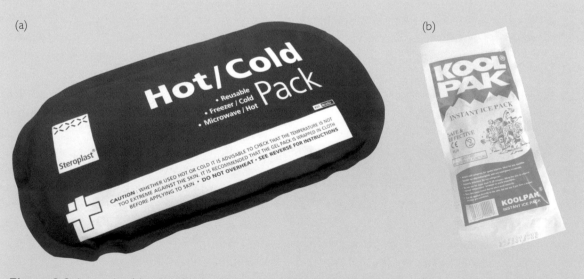

Figure 2.2 Ice packs: (a) reuseable hot/cold pack (b) instant ice pack

Here, we use a standard cotton crepe bandage and wrap it around the limb, altering the pressure as we do so. To increase the pressure still further, a layer of cotton wool may be placed over the bandage and a second layer of bandage applied. This type of bandage is used in hospitals for poor circulation in the legs, for example, and following certain types of knee surgery.

- **Elevation** is used to avoid swelling from fluid pooling through the pull of gravity. Swelling should normally be removed via the lymphatic vessels, but these may be overwhelmed after injury. In addition, the return of the circulation towards the heart (venous return) is helped by muscle contraction – a feature called the *accessory muscle pump*. As blood vessels travel through muscle, the rhythmical contraction and relaxation of muscles creates a pumping mechanism to assist the blood flowing up through the legs. Following injury the enforced rest removes this feature, and the combination of poor blood circulation and reduced lymph flow alters the fluid balance in the legs. By elevating the legs the effects of gravity are reduced. Simply putting the foot up on a stool while sitting will stop fluid pooling around the ankle. The circulation may be further helped if the limb is elevated above the level of the heart. In the sub-acute and chronic stages of an injury this may be achieved by lying on the ground with the legs resting on a stool or even with them resting vertically up against a wall. This encourages the flow of fluids from the feet towards the groin. Elevation may also be used at night by simply placing a cushion between the bed base and mattress at the foot end of the bed. Although the decline produced is quite small (5–10 degrees), because it remains for the whole night the effect can be quite significant, with ankle swelling reduced substantially by the morning.

Keypoint

Elevation may be applied in stages: (i) sitting with the foot up on a stool; (ii) lying on the floor with the feet up on a stool; and (iii) lying on the floor with the feet resting up against a wall.

SPORTS MASSAGE

One of the most useful treatment tools you have is sports massage. This may be applied either to yourself or using a partner. Massage is simply a modification of stroking which parents instinctively use on children and rubbing which we all instinctively do when we knock into something. The effects on the body are through two mechanisms. First, massage stimulates nerves (*see* chapter 1) to reduce pain and help relax muscle spasm. Second, the pressure used in massage causes tissue changes, moving fluids and moulding the tissues like kneading bread.

Before you practise massage there is some preparation you need to do. Hygiene is important because massage presses material into the skin, and any dirt can irritate or infect the skin. Make sure your partner has a shower before massage; as well as cleaning the skin it will help to relax their muscles and improve blood flow to the skin. Never massage someone who has just come off the sports field covered in mud or from the gym very sweaty.

Wash your hands and make sure your fingernails are short and smooth. Take off rings, watches and jewellery.

> ## Keypoint
>
> Hygiene is vital prior to massage. Never massage someone with mud or sweat on the skin – ask them to shower first. Wash your hands, keep your nails short and remove watches and jewellery.

Have your partner undress to shorts and bra and lie down on an exercise mat on the floor. Have a large bath towel to hand to cover up the parts of their body which have just been massaged, to keep them warm. Place a cushion beneath their feet to relax the thighs, and either get them to place their hands beneath their forehead or put a folded towel under their forehead, to stop them squashing their nose. It is important for them to relax, and if any part of their body is pressing into the floor painfully, their muscles will go into spasm.

Use some oil on your hands. This can be a ready-made aromatherapy oil or simply a sterile oil from the chemist (*see* fig 2.3). Use enough oil for your hands to glide across their skin (slip) without creating skin drag, but not too much, as some of the movements will involve lifting the skin (grip). Experience will tell you the correct amount of oil to use to combine both slip and grip. Rather than oil you may choose a specially made massage gel or cream. These are liquefying creams which get thinner as they warm up (*see* fig 2.3).

Kneel beside your partner, making sure that you have a pad beneath your knees for comfort. Some

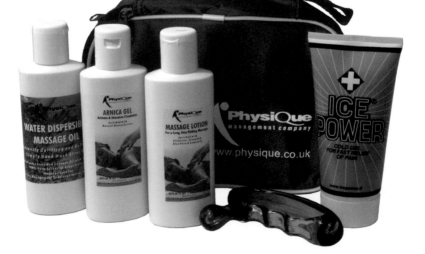

Figure 2.3 (a) Massage supplies – water dispersible oil, massage gel, massage lotion, massage tool (index knobber) and cooling gel

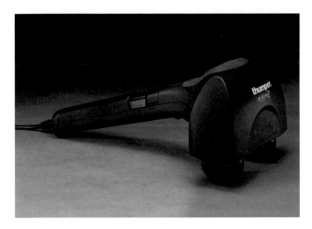

Figure 2.4 Example of a mechanical massage machine

the end of the stoke, release the pressure and relax your hand as you return it to the start position. In this way your hand and arm get a chance to recover between strokes. Perform 3–5 repetitions of the stroke on one part of the skin before moving onto another, aiming to cover the whole body area. The direction of the stoke is always towards the centre of the chest, so foot to thigh or hand to shoulder. This is the direction in which the lymph fluid flows through its vessels towards the heart. Where swelling is very bad, massage the upper part of the limb first (knee to thigh) to clear these lymph channels, before massaging the lower part (foot to knee).

people like to kneel on both knees (high kneeling), others on just one knee with the other foot flat on the floor (half kneeling). If you have access to a massage couch, so much the better. These are foldable trestle tables made of either wood or aluminium. The legs fold down flat and the couch folds in half to contain the legs, leaving an easily stored suitcase shape – a good investment if you are going to use massage regularly (*see* fig 2.5).

There are four categories of movements, some traditionally described using French names:

- **Stroking** (effleurage) is performed with the flat of your hands (*see* fig 2.6, page 16). Rather than pressing with your hand, lean forwards slightly, keeping your elbows locked, and press into the skin. To avoid digging into the skin, either keep your fingers straight and massage in line with the fingers, or contour the limb with your hand and lead with the side of your hand or web space. Press evenly and move slowly, as though you were pressing oil from a sponge. As you get to

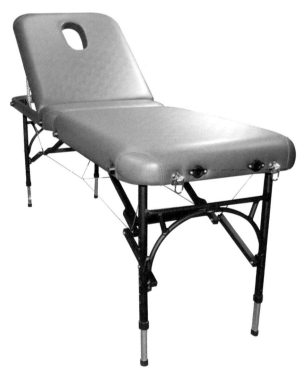

Figure 2.5 A typical portable massage couch – the legs fold up into the base and the whole couch folds into two sections to form a suitcase shape

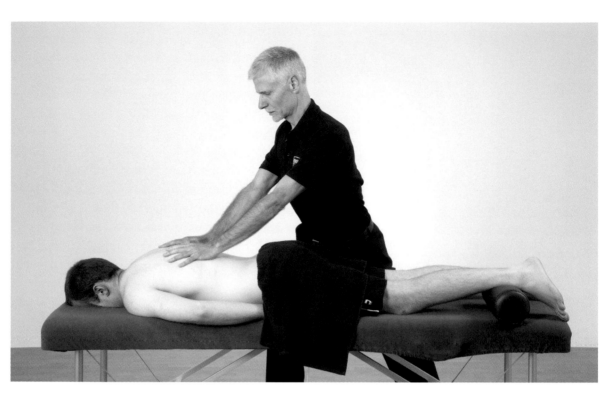

Figure 2.6 Stroking (effleurage)

Keypoint

When using a deep stroking massage (effleurage) to relieve swelling in the leg, massage the portion of the limb closest to the body (proximal) first to clear fluid from the lymphatic vessels. The tissue area further from the body (distal) is massaged second.

- **Lifting and rolling or wringing actions** (petrissage) are performed by lightly gripping the skin and lifting it up. Lift with the whole of your hand, not just your fingertips as this can pinch the skin painfully. A wringing action (*see* fig 2.7, page 17) is performed by lifting the skin and underlying muscle. Once lifted, move your hands forwards and backwards against each other to form an 'S' shape with the tissues. Release, move the hands to the next tissue section and repeat. Rolling and wringing (*see* fig 2.8, page 18) lifts the skin without the underlying muscle. Now, the roll of skin may be moved by pressing the hands forwards across the skin surface so that the skin roll moves like a wave. Both wringing and rolling encourage one area of tissue to move on another and so form an action called *tissue mobilisation*.

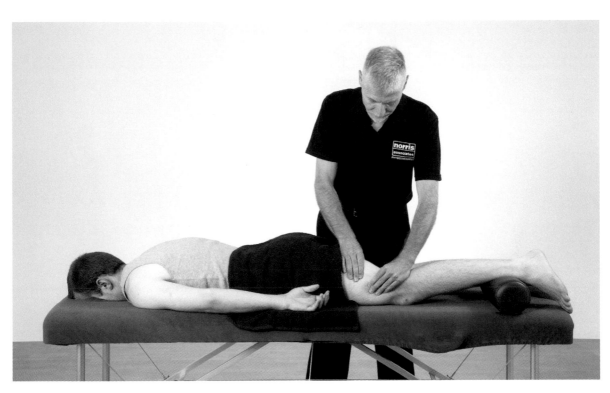

Figure 2.7 Wringing (petrissage)

Keypoint

Tissue mobilisation is performed when one section of tissue is moved on another. The effect is to encourage free movement of the tissue and may be used after injury or a heavy workout where waste products have built up in the tissues.

- **Striking actions** (tapotement) are used to stimulate the skin. The skin becomes red as blood flows into the area, and nerve fibres are stimulated, easing pain and stiffness. Strike the skin with either your fingertips (mild), the sides of your hands (heavier) (*see* fig 2.9, page 19) or side of the open fist (intense). Striking actions are used over fleshy areas such as the back of the thigh, but not over bony areas such as the outside of the shin. Try to get a rhythm going slowly to begin with, but as you become more practised you can speed up. The secret is to release your wrists so that your arms provide the power for the massage movement, and your hands, being the massage tool, simply transmit the force that the arms have created. As you move across the body ease off the pressure as you approach thinner or more delicate regions. For example, if you are

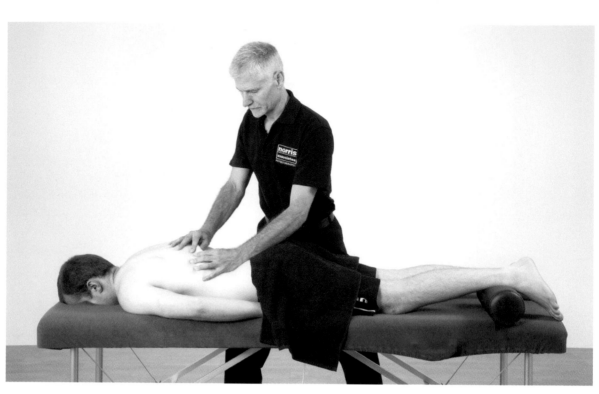

Figure 2.8 Rolling

massaging the thigh, the striking action eases as you get close to the knee and is not performed at all over the kneecap (patella).

- **Frictional movements** (or *frictions*) are a to-and-fro action. Using a light touch the fingers move across the skin surface, but with a heavier touch the skin and finger moves as one unit, so it is the muscle beneath which receives the force of the massage. This deeper action is often performed across the fibres of a muscle by physiotherapists and is called a *deep transverse friction* (DTF). Frictions may also be performed in a circular fashion – a technique particularly useful on areas of dense swelling around a joint.

For example, after an ankle sprain (*see* chapter 4) a pocket of firm swelling often remains below the outer ankle bone (lateral malleolus). Circular frictional massage may be used to break up the swelling and encourage the body to reabsorb the fluid.

A variety of mechanical massage machines are available (*see* fig 2.4, page 15). These generally produce different intensities of vibration. The contact area (head) of the machine usually comes in a variety of shapes and sizes to access large or small body areas. Although not as variable or specific as using your own hands, a massage machine can be useful in cases where there is a large amount of swelling or

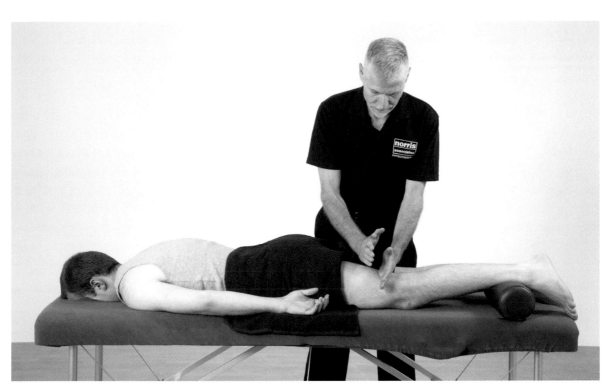

Figure 2.9 Striking actions (tapotement) – using the sides of the hands

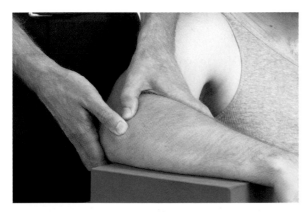

Figure 2.10 Frictions

where muscle spasm is intense. In each case the firm massage required will be very taxing on your

hands, so to begin the massage using a machine can reduce your workload.

TAPING

Taping or strapping is a method of supporting a joint, limiting movement of an area, or of re-educating a movement where an action is faulty.

TYPES

Taping is general categorised as *structural* or *functional*. Structural taping *limits movement* and protects a joint. This is the type you would use to support your ankle after a sprain, for example, and is fairly strong when applied. When you sprain your ankle it is the outside (lateral) ligament which is typically injured. This ligament helps protect the ankle joint from moving inwards too far. Because this ligament has torn during injury, the taping must protect this inward ankle movement. Strips of tape are applied to limit the inward ankle movement while allowing free movement in other directions.

Functional taping does not limit movement, but helps to guide it. An example of a functional tape is that used for back pain (*see* chapter 8), where tape strips are placed either side of the spine to discourage too much forward bending. Although it would be possible to bend with the taping on, the tape gives feedback as it tightens and pulls on the skin when you bend, supporting the area.

MATERIALS

Several materials are available (*see* table 2.1) and it is often useful to put these together in a bag (*see* fig 2.3, page 14) if you look after a team for example. *Elastic tape* contours to the body and expands slightly as muscles contract. It is used to compress, for example where swelling is likely to form. In addition, it can also be used to support a muscle, where it is placed pre-stretched onto the skin. As it recoils it provides a firm compression of a flat area. *Non-elastic tape* (also called *zinc oxide*) is used to limit movement of a joint and support an area more firmly. Because it is non-elastic, this type of tape can cut into the skin if put on too tightly. All adhesive tapes stick directly to the skin and so there are a number of precautions. Skin to be taped should be clean. If the skin surface is very hairy, either it should be shaved or an *underwrap* used. Where shaved, a skin preparation lotion (skin prep) is normally applied to prevent skin irritation. Underwrap is a thin sponge tape which wraps around the limb before non-elastic taping is applied. It protects skin against movement of the tape, which can irritate the skin surface. *Cohesive tape* is rigid tape which is thinner and lighter than adhesive tape. It is coated with an adherent material rather than an adhesive, meaning that the tape sticks only to itself and not to the skin. Cohesive tape can be reused a number of times and is water-resistant. Where a joint has a prominent piece of bone (ankle or knee for example), this may be protected by a *gel* or *foam pad*. In addition *felt* material may be cut to shape and used to fill spaces around the ankle, for example.

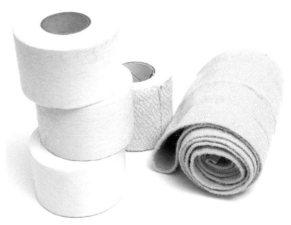

Figure 2.11 Types of taping (left to right): non-elastic, cohesive, elastic

Definition

Adhesive tape has a type of glue on the back which will stick directly to your skin. *Adherent tape* has a tacky chemical backing which sticks to itself but not to your skin.

Table 2.1	Taping supplies
Material	**Description**
Rigid tape	Also called **zinc oxide**. Normally has a serrated edge for ease of tearing and comes in various widths (1.25 mm, 25 mm, 38 mm, 50 mm).
Elastic tape	Generally comes in 4.5 m length and various widths (25 mm, 50 mm, 75 mm).
Cohesive tape	Crinkle fabric which conforms to the body surface and tears easily, available in 50 mm and 75 mm widths. Non-slip and water-resistant.
Crepe bandage	Traditional cotton nursing bandage. Non-adhesive and reusable. Must be secured with safety pins or adhesive tape strips.
Underwrap	Sponge rubber tape on a roll.
Padding	Felt or foam sheets in several thicknesses. Cut to shape.
Gel skin protector	Single sheets of gel back plastic.
Cotton wool sheet	Sheet of cotton wool on a roll.
Adhesive spray	Light adhesive in a spray can.
Adhesive remover	Available in a bottle or as an individual sachet.
Skin prep	Spray-on or available in a bottle.
Petroleum jelly	To protect prominent bones.
Razor	Either an electric clipper or a safety razor to remove hair.
Scissors	Blunt-ended to cut tape but avoid piercing the skin.
Tape cutter	V-shaped end containing a single safety blade.
Sterile gloves	To be used wherever the skin is damaged, to avoid contamination with body fluids (lymph, blood).

TECHNIQUE

Taping may be applied either *continuously* or in *strips*. For continuous taping, the end of the tape is attached to the skin and the tape roll is unwound as the taping is applied. Where tape strips are used, initially an anchor is applied (*see* fig 4.2, page 42). The anchor forms a firm base to attach further tape strips. Normally two anchors are used with tape reins running between the two. Several reins are used contouring the body part to build up a secure application. A fixing strip is then used to hold the tape application in place. Figure 4.2 also shows a continuous taping sequence for a typical ankle sprain (lateral ligament tear). Figure 2.12 (overleaf) shows tape strip application for low back pain. Other examples of specific tapings are shown in the chapters dealing with individual injuries.

COLD

We have seen that cold in the form of an ice pack is used as part of sports first aid within the PRICE mnemonic. Cold may also used therapeutically later on in the rehabilitation phase in the form of ice massage and contrast bathing. Ice baths may also be used both to treat an injury and to aid recovery.

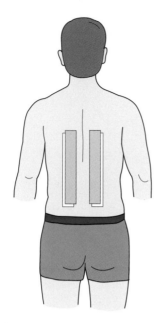

Figure 2.12 Example of functional taping

Ice massage is used to relieve pain and give a local numbing effect as well as to increase local blood flow. To perform ice massage you need to hold an ice cube, a situation made considerably more comfortable by freezing water inside a polystyrene cup and peeling off the top of it to expose the ice. Gripping onto the insulated polystyrene cup is easier than gripping a slippery frozen ice cube. Commercial available equivalents include the ice-up massager. As the ice will melt during treatment, make sure you put the body area to be treated on a towel or plastic sheet to catch the ice water trickling off the skin. Place some oil or lotion on the skin to protect the skin surface. Touch the ice to the skin using light pressure, resting rather than pressing onto the skin. The massage action is a slow circular motion covering the area of pain. Make sure that you keep the ice moving: if you stop for too long the procedure

becomes painful and eventually the skin may blister.

> ### Keypoint
> When performing ice massage, keep the ice moving. If you stop, the area can become painful and an ice burn may result.

Contrast bathing is used over larger areas of swelling, especially the ankle and hand. For this you will need two bowls. Fill one with hot water. This should be comfortably hot but not scalding. Fill the other bowl with cold water and place some ice cubes in it. Put your foot into the hot water and then the cold water. After a time both bowls begin to change to the same temperature, so it is a good idea to have some spare ice cubes ready to top up the cold water bowl and a jug of hot water to top up the hot one. Table 2.2 shows suggested timings for contrast bathing, but, remember, the procedure must be comfortable and not painful. The regimen gradually builds up the time of each immersion before changing to the other bowl. The total immersion time of the session is also increased. Aim to spend longer in the cold water, and build up the amount of time you spend using the technique. It is useful to perform gentle toe and ankle movements while your foot is in the water, as this additionally helps to reduce swelling and ease fluid congestion. Perform each contrast bathing session in the morning and afternoon (twice daily), or in the morning, afternoon and evening (3 times daily), giving a total of five days bathing. Rest on day six and repeat as required.

Table 2.2	Contrast bathing regimen				
	Session 1	**Session 2**	**Session 3**	**Session 4**	**Session 5**
Cold (10–15°C)	2 min	3 min	4 min	4 min	5 min
Hot (35–40°C)	0.5 min	1 min	1 min	1 min	2 min
Total time	10 min	10 min	12 min	15 min	18–20 min

Note: Each session is practised twice or three times daily. Take a rest day after session 5.

Ice baths are often used by professional sports clubs for injury rehab and recovery from competition. An ice bath automatically cools the water and has a whirlpool setting which circulates the iced water around the body part to enhance the bathing effect. One of the problems with intense exercise is that the body tissues become less efficient if they overheat, which they often do during intense endurance activities. Cooling the body tissues prolongs the period of efficient exercise before overheating occurs. Ice baths can therefore be used to pre-cool the body prior to competition. At half-time during a game ice baths can aid short-term recovery; after a game they aid recovery and reduce stiffness, meaning that an athlete is ready to compete again earlier.

Ice baths work by cooling the skin and reducing skin blood flow. As less blood flows to the skin, more can remain in the muscles to help sports performance. In addition, more blood remains within the body organs and it is these that are responsible for detoxing after exercise and removing the waste products produced by working muscles.

HEAT

Heat may be applied via heat lamps which shine heat onto your skin (*radiant heating*) and packs which are in direct contact with your skin (*conduction heating*). Two types of lamps are generally used: *infrared* (visible) and *radiant heat* (invisible). Infrared lamps have bulbs which are red on the end and shine red light onto the skin. As well as heating the area, the visible red light is relaxing and easily directed onto a body area. Radiant heat lamps have a ceramic and metal heating unit rather than a bulb. The heat that they produce is invisible and more intense than that produced by the bulb of an infrared lamp. In addition, radiant heat lamps (also called *black lamps*) take time to warm up and are more difficult to direct as their heat rays cannot be seen.

The heat from a lamp will only penetrate 3–5 mm into the skin, but in so doing will cause blood to flow into the area – the body's response to try to cool down. You will notice that your skin is red (erythema) when the lamp has been on for a while. The heat helps stimulate nerve endings in your skin to relieve pain and reduce muscle spasm. These effects are useful prior to massage for example.

Heat packs usually contain gel or granules (often grain such as wheat or barley). The gel packs are generally heated in hot water or a microwave, while the grain can only be microwaved. The grain packs actually absorb a small amount of moisture from the atmosphere and so provide a moist heat. A normal hot water bottle may also be used, or just hot water from a shower or bath.

23

Although heat is useful to relax an area, ease stiffness and reduce pain, there are two concerns. First, heat may burn. You should *never* apply a heat lamp without supervision. If you relax too much and go to sleep you can give yourself a very bad burn. Second, a heat pack should only ever be placed *on* yourself. Do not lie on a pack, as the heat combined with pressure can burn. Although the heat from a lamp will build up over time, a pack will cool down and so is safer over time.

Keypoint

Do not apply a heat lamp without supervision. If you go to sleep with the lamp on, you can give yourself a very serious burn requiring hospital treatment.

CREAMS, LOTIONS, RUBS

A huge variety of creams and lotions are available to the sports person. Generally these are divided into three categories (*see* table 2.3). Some creams feel warm or cold, but be cautious because this is a skin nerve (sensory) effect rather than true cooling or heating. If you want to cool an area after injury, use ice; if you want the benefits of heating on the tissues, use a hot pack. The creams will give a temporary feeling and can be useful short term, but not over a prolonged period. Creams may also have aromatherapy oils within them. These oils have small enough molecules to go through the skin and have therapeutic effects. Similarly, creams and lotions may contain medical drugs used to reduce pain and inflammation. These should be bought from a pharmacist, who will advise on effect and importantly any interactions with other drugs that are being taken or medical conditions.

Table 2.3	Creams and lotions
Type	**Effect**
Heating and cooling	Contain chemicals which irritate the skin to cause a heating (rubefacient) or cooling (cryothermal) effect. Often given a colour and smell to associate with their effect: heating creams are generally red, while cooling ones are blue.
Aromatherapy	Contain essential oils, such as camomile and orange. The oils are absorbed into the skin to give a therapeutic effect.
Medical	Contain a drug, such as salicylic acid to aid pain relief and reduce swelling.

Terms you should know:

Accessory muscle pump – squeezing of blood vessels which pass through the leg muscles to help blood return to the heart.

Conduction heating – heat applied through contact with the body.

Contrast bathing – alternately heating and cooling a limb by immersion.

Cryothermal – having a cooling effect.

Functional rest – resting an injured tissue but continuing to exercise on uninjured parts of the body.

Infrared heat lamp – heating source which shines visible red light onto the body.

Metabolic rate – the speed of chemical reactions in the body tissues.

Radiant heat lamp (black lamp) – invisible heat source.

Rubefacient – having a heating effect.

Underwrap – adhesive mesh put on the skin before other tape to protect the skin from irritation.

STRUCTURING
// REHABILITATION

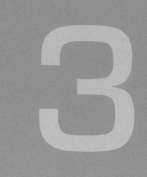

We have seen in chapter 1 how your tissues heal, and in chapter 2 some of the methods you can use to help this healing process as part of sports injuries treatment. Now, we will look closely at how we can structure a rehabilitation programme to get you back to sport quickly and effectively.

WORKING WITH HEALING

In chapter 2 we saw that healing involves the formation of a bridge across damaged tissue. The bridge begins immediately after injury as a blood clot which gradually shrinks and is replaced by fibrous tissue. Initially, the fibres of this new tissue are arranged in a haphazard way. This fibre arrangement is quite weak and known as a *disorganised format*. Gradually, the fibres realign in the direction that they are stressed and become organised. This fibre realignment process is dependent on movement, but this movement must match the stage of healing. Too much movement in terms of either volume or intensity in the early stages of healing will cause the fibrous tissue bridge to break down.

As healing progresses, the tissue bridge becomes stronger and more able to handle the stresses and strains of exercise. It is now essential to stress the tissue enough for it to strengthen

Definition
Training intensity is how hard an exercise is (e.g. how much weight is lifted) and *training volume* is how much exercise you do (e.g. sets and repetitions).

correctly. Too little stress on the tissue during the later stages of healing when the tissue is remodelling (*see* chapter 1) will result in it being weak. This is similar to exercising in the gym. To build strength, you need to stress your muscles using the resistance of weight or bands. If the resistance is too light, your strength will not improve. The same is true during rehabilitation.

We saw in chapter 1 that healing moves forwards continuously, but for convenience can be divided into three phases. During these three phases the strength of the healing tissue changes. Initially during injury, tissues have torn or been bruised so their strength rapidly reduces from normal. In this phase (acute) we must protect the damaged tissues from further injury and so exercise is not used – we say it is *contraindicated*. As the tissues begin to heal, a blood clot forms and shrinks, so, although the tissue is changing, it is still weak and easily disrupted by movement. This represents the *lag phase* (*see* fig 3.1). Although time has passed since you were injured and the tissues have begun to heal, tissue strength has not changed at all. Exercise remains contraindicated until about 24–48 hours after injury. The time variation is dependent on the size of the injury.

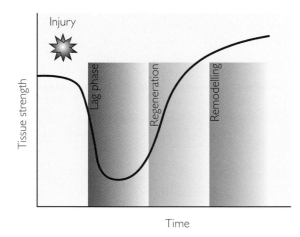

Figure 3.1 Phases of healing

After this time we progress to the next stage of healing (sub-acute), where the blood clot is being replaced by fibrous tissue and we enter the phase of *regeneration* – as fresh tissue grows the area gradually becomes stronger. As tissue strength increases, the amount of exercise you are able to use can increase. It is important that the pace of increase in exercise matches the increasing tissue strength. Too much and the new tissue can break down and re-injure; too little and the new tissue will be weak.

Tissue strength continues to increase until we reach a point where no new tissue is formed. From now on tissue strength slows, and the tissue begins to change to match that which existed prior to injury. This phase is *remodelling*, which occurs 4–6 weeks after the injury. Fibrous tissue never exactly matches the original which it has replaced, but, importantly, full function will return with correct rehabilitation.

EXERCISE PROGRESSION

How do we match the rate of exercise increase with the changing strength of the healing tissue? The key here is feedback from your injury. You must continually monitor the effect exercise is having on your injury – in short, listen to your body and keep listening. At no time should you exercise through increasing pain. When you begin rehabilitation you are exercising a part of the body which has been injured and not moved for some time. It is inevitable that you will feel some pain, but we need to spend some time looking more closely at this.

MONITOR DISCOMFORT AND PAIN

When something is painful, OK it hurts, but how much? Rather than say 'a little' or 'a lot', we can use a hospital-based pain scale (officially called a *numerical rating scale*). This is a score from 0 (no pain) to 10 (maximum pain) (*see* fig 3.2, overleaf). Aim to monitor what you feel in an injured body part throughout your rehabilitation programme. First, pain should not increase, and second, the intensity of the pain should not be great. Pain intensity (how painful the injury feels) should be no higher than 5 or 6 on the pain scale. If it is higher than this, reduce the intensity of the exercise. If you are lifting weights, for example, use less weight or perform fewer repetitions. As you exercise, if pain is caused by stiffness and new tissue stretching out, the pain should reduce with activity. You may score 6 for the first 2 or 3 repetitions and this might reduce to 4 or 5 as you get into the exercise. After a rest, when you perform your second set of an exercise, the pain may once more reduce. This is a sign that the tissue is reacting in a positive way to the exercise and you can continue. However, if your pain score begins at 5 or 6 and increases to 7 or 8, you must stop immediately. Do not finish your set. Rest and try again. If the pain stays at 5 or 6 and does not increase, you can continue, but cautiously. Increasing pain means that you are putting too much stress on the healing tissues and they are likely to break down. Your aim should be to stress the tissues to get them to change positively (adapt) by becoming stronger or more flexible. If pain is increasing, the tissue is changing negatively (maladaption): it may be tearing or becoming inflamed. Either way you are interfering with the healing process and risking a significant setback.

Keypoint

Do not exercise through increasing pain – stop immediately, rest and try again. If pain still increases, abandon the exercise.

OVERLOAD THE TISSUE

To be effective, exercise must challenge the body tissue – this challenge is called *overload*. When the body is overloaded, tissue breaks down at a microscopic level and rebuilds itself to become stronger – a process called *supercompensation*. To achieve this, exercise must challenge the body to a greater extent than day-to-day activities. For example, if we perform an arm curl exercise, the action (elbow flexion) is similar to picking up a teacup. We would not expect to strengthen the arm bending muscle (biceps) by picking up a teacup because, although the action is the same, the overload is not great enough.

Overload is made up of four factors described by the mnemonic FITT, standing for *Frequency, Intensity, Time* and *Type*.

- **Frequency** is how often you practise an exercise, for example twice each day or three times each week.

- **Intensity** is how hard an exercise is. In strength training this is normally measured in comparison to the maximum weight you can lift once (1 repetition maximum or 1RM); with stretching it is the how far you stretch as a

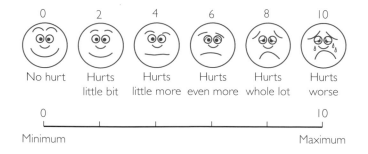

Figure 3.2 Pain scale

proportion of your maximum range of movement (ROM), for example 60% max ROM or 80% max ROM.

- **Time** is the duration of the exercise, for example running for 20 minutes or 1 hour. It also refers to the duration of a repetition, for example using a very slow action (superslow technique) in weight training to emphasise muscle contraction.

- **Type** is the category of exercise, such as strength training, aerobics, stretching or plyometrics. Each of these can be subdivided depending on which of the 'S' factors of fitness are worked (*see* below).

These four overload factors are called *training variables* (*see* table 3.1), and altering any of them will change the overall work intensity. The total amount of work is often expressed in sets and repetitions, and together the description of an exercise using these variables is commonly referred to as *training volume*.

For example, heavy weight training is clearly harder than light jogging (exercise type), while slow walking is easier than fast walking (intensity). Performing a trunk curl exercise every hour throughout the day is harder than performing it every other day (frequency), and doing 10 repetitions is easier than 100 repetitions

Keypoint
Training volume is the total amount of work performed during an exercise by combining the training variables frequency, intensity, time and type.

(duration). Performing the trunk curl everyday for 3 sets of 10 repetitions gives a larger training volume than performing it three times each week for 2 sets of 12 repetitions.

PROGRESS THE EXERCISE

You have seen that you need to overload tissue to enhance its performance. As the tissue improves, exercise must get harder to continue to challenge the tissue sufficiently. This structured increase in hardness of exercise is called *progression*. Most people think of progressing weight training by increasing the weight lifted and progressing running by running further or faster. In fact there are several ways to progress an exercise and the one we choose will depend on the injury, stage of healing and tissue condition. Table 3.2 shows some methods of exercise progression and, although you will not use each factor with every exercise, let's spend some time briefly explaining

Table 3.1	Training variables
Variable	**Meaning**
Type	Exercise category (weight training, stretching etc.)
Duration	How long exercise lasts
Frequency	How often exercise is practiced (daily, weekly etc.)
Intensity	How hard exercise is

29

Table 3.2	Factors to consider when progressing exercise
• Leverage • Stability and base of support • Energy systems • Momentum • Friction • Speed of movement	• Complexity • Gravity • Muscle work • Range of motion • Starting position • Resistance

how they work. We will see illustrations of each factor in the clinical chapters 4–12.

- **Leverage** progresses an exercise by increasing the weight (load) of an object being lifted. Its effective weight is greatest when the body part performing the lift gets closer to the horizontal and lessens as it gets further away from the horizontal (*see* fig 3.3). In figure 3.3a, the person is lifting a dumbbell out sideways. The leverage increases as their arm gets closer to the horizontal and so the exercise is harder at this point. By lying on their side (*see* fig 3.3b) they perform the same movement, but now as the arm is lifted it is gradually moving away from the horizontal and so the movement is getting

easier. This exercise is therefore harder (a progression) in the standing position than in the lying position.

- **Stability and base of support** becomes more important in balance exercises. Standing on one leg can be an important exercise during the rehabilitation of an ankle injury (*see* chapter 4). Stability is harder to maintain when the base of support is narrower. This means that a standing exercise performed with the legs apart is easier (therefore, more stable) than one performed with the legs together, and this in turn is easier than one performed standing on one leg (*see* fig 3.4, page 31).

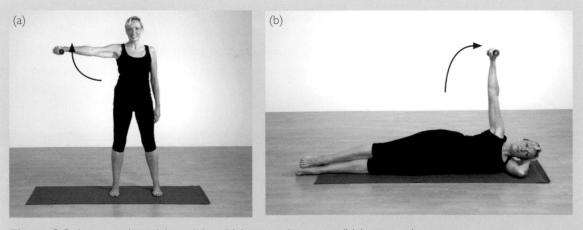

Figure 3.3 Leverage in weight training: (a) leverage increases; (b) leverage decreases

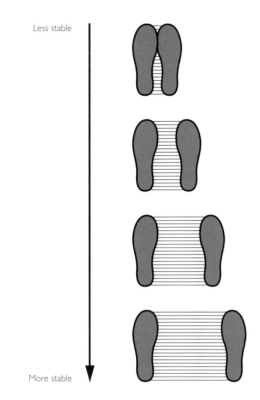

Less stable

More stable

Figure 3.4 Changing base of support and stability

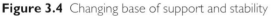

and they are getting fitter. However, if they were a long jumper, who requires short intense sprints, the training would not match their sport (*see* training specificity, page 36). We would be training the athlete aerobically (5-mile run), while they needed anaerobic training (repetitions of short sprints).

- **Momentum** is important when performing faster actions. Momentum builds up if you move your arm quickly, for example, meaning that it is difficult to stop moving suddenly. The heavier a limb is, the more momentum it will have, so holding a dumbbell will increase momentum. Momentum is important at the very start of rehab and at the very end. At the start, a very stiff joint can often be freed up by using very gentle swinging actions of the limb. At the end of rehab, the ability of muscle to work quickly enough to control momentum is important when performing cutting drills (changing direction rapidly) in sports such as football and rugby.

- **Energy systems** refers to how the energy to perform an exercise is created by the body. Broadly speaking there are two ways. First, with oxygen (aerobic): a method used for long runs and endurance events. Second, without oxygen (anaerobic): a method used for short, hard training such as sprints and weight lifting.

  It is important to use the same energy system in rehabilitation as will be required eventually in sport. For example, in rehab a runner may begin by running ¼ mile and build up to ½ mile and eventually 5 miles. We can see that the exercise is getting harder (progressing)

- **Friction** may be used to progress an exercise in the same way as increasing weight or using a thicker exercise band. Often the resistance setting on home-user static cycles are friction-based using either mechanical or electromagnetic braking. Friction can also be used for sliding. Slide training actions can be performed using a pair of thick socks on a shiny surface. In this case friction is reduced to allow free movement, for example side-to-side leg actions. Increasing friction can be used for running using a rope attached around the waist connected to a car tyre. The friction of the tyre pulled over a sports pitch significantly increases the difficulty of running.

- **Complexity** of an exercise is important for coordination. A simpler exercise should be used initially as it is easier to understand, control and correct. Gradually, as confidence is gained, more complex actions are used.

- **Speed of movement** ties up with momentum. Faster movements have greater momentum and are therefore more difficult to stop and control. They often use a different type of muscle work, relying partially on the elastic recoil of tissues. In addition, faster movements in some cases can be more complex to control, requiring greater concentration.

- **Gravity** is used as part of leverage as we have seen above. Another use of gravity is in the early stages of rehab, when you can use it to free off a stiff joint or to ease back pain. Allowing the arm to hang freely while performing a shoulder exercise (*see* chapter 10) is an excellent way to begin an exercise which would otherwise be painful. Hanging from a high bar and allowing gravity to stretch the spine can relieve compression and pain in the low back (*see* chapter 8).

- **Muscle work** is carried out not just to lift an object, but also to hold it still and lower it under control. The lifting action is an example of a concentric muscle contraction, holding is isometric and lowering under control is eccentric.

  The three types of muscle work can be further illustrated when standing up and sitting down in a chair. As you stand up, your thigh muscles are tightening and working concentrically. If you stop yourself just short of full standing and hold the position, the same muscles work isometrically. As you slowly lower yourself down again back into the chair, the muscles are working eccentrically.

  In general the order of strength reduces from eccentric to isometric and finally concentric. You can illustrate this using a simple chin-up exercise on a bar. When you feel you can perform no more chins, step onto a bench and hold yourself with your elbows bent to 90 degrees. You will find that you can do this (isometric hold) although you cannot lift yourself anymore (concentric). Finally, when you can no longer hold yourself, you will find that you may be able to squeeze out a couple more repetitions if your training partner lifts you up and you lower yourself slowly (eccentric). This is a frequently used technique in bodybuilding known as *forced repetitions*.

- **Range of motion** is how far you are able to move a joint (*see* fig 3.5, page 33). Normally, throughout the day you only use a limited amount of movement in your joints because you will rarely open (extend) or close (flex) the joint fully (*see* fig 3.5a). This middle part of the joint's movement is called *mid range* (*see* fig 3.5d). When you fully open a joint you are moving it to *outer range* and when you fully close it you are moving to its *inner range* (*see* fig 3.5c). The key during rehab is both to use full range movements during training and to match the movement range with that used in the sport an athlete will return to. For example, after an elbow injury (*see* chapter 11) you may be giving arm exercise to a javelin thrower. Because the

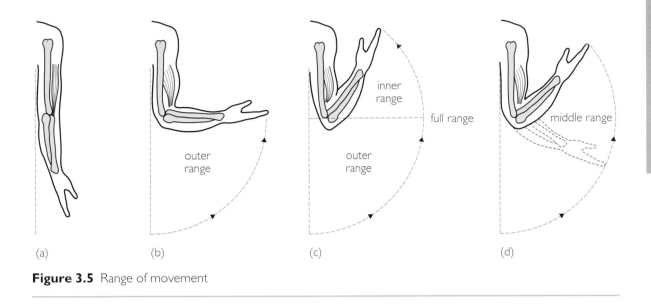

(a) (b) (c) (d)

Figure 3.5 Range of movement

elbow was injured there is a temptation to protect the joint and avoid full range movement. In the final stages of rehab, however, to prepare the athlete fully before competing, it is essential that they train the elbow to full outer range to mimic the stress on the joint which will be encountered when they throw the javelin.

- **Starting position**, as the term suggests, is the position in which an athlete starts an exercise. This should be both comfortable and safe so that they feel confident to exercise on a body part which was previously injured and may still be painful. Often, using the same exercise but varying the starting position is an excellent way of creating variety in a workout. Because the exercise used is essentially the same, it makes learning far easier.

- **Resistance** can be provided by several methods. Weights, bands, pulleys and water are all methods of providing resistance. To progress an exercise, resistance must increase gradually and keep pace with healing. Again, using different methods of resistance creates variety and prevents staleness and boredom during rehabilitation.

SELECT APPROPRIATE EXERCISE COMPONENTS

We talk about strength exercise and stretching exercise as though each was completely separate. The fact is that very few exercises are completely pure and most have a variety of individual components. So, for example, the bench press exercise is categorised as a strength movement, but it also stretches the chest. For some individuals it may be better to reduce the weight (strength focus) and simply use a wooden pole to perform the action, making sure that the bar goes onto the chest completely (stretch focus). To categorise an exercise we must determine each component of

Table 3.3	Components of an exercise – the 'S' factors
• Stamina	Cardiopulmonary and local muscle endurance
• Suppleness	Range of motion (ROM), static/dynamic flexibility
• Strength	Concentric/isometric/eccentric
• Spirit	Psychological aspects of fitness/injury
• Speed	Rate/reaction time
• Skill	Coordination/ proprioception/agility
• Specificity	Specific adaptation to imposed demand (SAID)

the exercise: for convenience these can be described as 'S' factors (*see* table 3.3).

Stamina refers to both cardiopulmonary and local muscle endurance. Local muscle endurance is important in holding exercises and stability training. Cardiopulmonary fitness, the type used in aerobic training, is important to restore following injury, as further injury can occur when a person becomes fatigued towards the end of the game.

Suppleness (or flexibility) training is important to rehabilitation and vital to sporting performance. However, it is important to realise that there are several types of stretching. These include static (hold), dynamic (movement) and PNF (reflex) stretching. For further details on stretching see *The Complete Guide to Stretching* (3rd edition) by Christopher Norris published by A&C Black (2007).

Strength includes concentric, eccentric and isometric varieties. All are important components of an exercise and it is essential that the type of strength training matches the precise requirements of a sport. For further details on strength training see *Bodytoning* by Christopher Norris published by A&C Black (2003).

The term *spirit* involves psychological factors which must be considered during rehabilitation. These are important to general training for both health and sports performance. Items such as motivation, how satisfied a person is with their own body, and a positive outlook on life fall into this category. The way a person reacts to injury also has psychological features depending on their psychological make-up and factors such as personality type and anxiety/stress levels. If an injury is severe or puts an athlete out of a major competition, there may be a large emotional reaction and the psychological state may be similar to that of grief encountered in life-threatening conditions (*see* table 3.4). In general, sports psychologists recognise three categories of response to injury in the athlete. Initially, the athlete becomes *injury-focused* and questions why and how the injury happened. This leads to *behaviour changes* and the athlete becomes agitated, feeling disbelief and often dwelling on self-pity. Finally athletes move through these phases and *accept* the injury. They begin to be positive, engaging in coping mechanisms. This later phase is where exercise is key as it gives the athlete the chance to participate in their own treatment.

Speed in this context also encompasses power. Speed is how fast we move (rate of movement), while power is how quickly we can move a resistance (rate of performing work); both are important for explosive actions in sport and vital components of the final stages of rehabilitation. Another aspect of speed is *muscle reaction time*.

Table 3.4	Similarity between emotional response to sports injury and a life-threatening condition
Denial	The unconscious refusal to accept facts: 'This cannot be happening to me, I've worked so hard in my training'; 'But I have a competition, I can't be injured now'.
Anger	Anger with themselves and others, making the athlete difficult to deal with: 'Who is to blame?'; 'They gave me the wrong exercise'; 'Those running shoes are to blame for this'.
Bargaining	Seek a compromise: 'Rather than rest, can I just run 3 miles instead of my normal 10?'; 'I'll go to the gym but I'll just use light weights – that will be OK won't it?'
Depression	Athlete withdraws and has long periods of silence: 'Just leave me alone'; 'What's the point?'
Acceptance	Athlete becomes emotionally detached from injury and becomes objective about recovery: 'I can't fight it, but I can work with it'.

This is how quickly you can contract a muscle and is especially important to joint stability. If we take an ankle sprain as an example (*see* chapter 4), the ligaments of the ankle have been overstretched and you need the muscles to compensate to keep your ankle stable on uneven surfaces. You can strengthen your ankle muscles using weight training, but this increased strength is of no use to you if your muscles do not contract quickly enough. For example, in the gym you may take 2 seconds to perform a heel raise action to strengthen your ankle. On rough ground, it may take only 0.25 seconds to sprain your ankle, so if you have only used weight training, your ankle muscles have not learned to contract quickly enough. Once you have strengthened your ankle muscles you don't need any more strength, but you do need to maintain the strength that you have and make your muscles contract more quickly. This is the function of speed training.

Skill is important to all actions, but especially those involving complex movements. Following injury, as we have seen in chapter 1, you can develop movement dysfunction, that is you move differently to avoid the pain of an injury and this becomes a habit. Remember, it is more important to regain movement quality before movement quantity, and this is especially the case with the complex skilled actions seen in sport. Failure to address skill can place stress on previously healthy body parts and cause fresh injury. If we use the example of the ankle injury we mentioned above, you will frequently walk with your ankle turning out after injury. If this change in walking is not corrected, it will place stress on the knee, hip and low back, eventually leading to pain in these parts of the body.

The final exercise component is *specificity*, which is dealt with below.

MATCH THE SPORT REQUIREMENTS

When a muscle is strengthened, its make-up actually changes. The muscle becomes larger and tighter, and there are alterations in the chemicals it contains. In addition, the way the brain controls the movement itself becomes smoother and more coordinated. All of these changes constitute what we call the *training adaptation*. In other words the changes which the body makes are a direct reaction to the training itself. The exact adaptation will closely reflect the type of exercise which has been used, and so we say that the muscle adaptation is *specific* to the demands placed upon it. A simple mnemonic to remember is SAID, standing for *Specific Adaptation to Imposed Demand*. The change in your body as a result of exercise (*adaptation*) will always closely match (be *specific* to) the exercise you use (the *imposed demand*).

An example from general sport may make this clearer. Imagine two people who run marathons. They want to reduce their times and go for a 'personal best'. If one person trains by running long distances and the other by running short sprints, who will be more successful in reducing their times? The answer is the person who runs distances. This type of training more accurately reflects the actions required during marathon running. Marathon runners need endurance. Short sprints will build mainly strength and speed, and so, although the person using sprint training is getting fitter, the fitness is not the type required for the final marathon race. His body has *adapted* but the changes do not closely match those needed for running the marathon: they are not truly *specific*.

Keypoint

For an exercise to be truly *specific* it must closely match the action which we hope to improve.

As another example let's look at the trunk. We need to know what function the trunk muscles perform and then tailor our training programme to improve this function. Trunk muscle function falls broadly into two categories: *support* (stabilisation), which is important after injury, and *movement*, which is more important to sports performance. During stabilisation the trunk muscles work mainly isometrically to make the trunk more solid. During movement the muscles work concentrically and eccentrically to perform actions such as bending and twisting. If you perform multiple sets of sit-ups you are actually working the movement function of the spine, rather than the stability function. This will have little effect on relieving pain as it not specific to your immediate injury needs and is more suited to later stage rehab.

So, for an exercise to be specific to a sport it must match the movements involved in that sport. We can also match an exercise to the general day-to-day requirements of our body. In this case the exercise is termed *functional*. For example, when you lift a heavy object such as a box you use your legs. We could argue that to strengthen your legs in the gym, using a leg extension machine would improve your ability to lift the box. However, although training on this machine will strengthen your legs, it does not rehearse the lifting action. Performing a deadlift action by lifting a barbell from the floor will also strengthen your leg muscles. In addition, the deadlift rehearses the correct method of lifting a heavy object from the floor. Because it mimics the action you will use when lifting a box each day, we say that the deadlift is a functional exercise, whereas the leg extension machine is a non-functional exercise.

> **Keypoint**
>
> A *functional* exercise mimics the day-to-day movements performed by a body part. It is 'real life' training.

CATEGORISING THE INJURY

When describing your sports injury it is useful to use standard descriptions as used by professional physiotherapists. This can be important for treatment records if you are involved with a sports team, for example, and will help when communicating with therapy professionals.

> **Keypoint**
>
> A ligament is *sprained*, a muscle *strained*. Each injury has a variety of categories reflecting the amount of tissue damage which has occurred.

SPRAINS AND STRAINS

A muscle is *strained* and a ligament *sprained*. Three grades of ligament injury can occur, depending on the intensity of the injury:

• **Grade (I)** ligament injury is a minor sprain with very little tissue damage. There will be moderate pain with some local swelling which forms gradually after injury and rests close to the injured area with little spread from here. You will be able to use the body part, but will find it a little painful to move the joint very far, or to move quickly.

• **Grade (II)** injury involves damage to more of the ligament fibres, and in some cases a portion of the ligament may detach from the bone. Swelling is far greater and accumulates more quickly. It will spread away from the injured area, settling around the joint. Pain is now intense, and it is very difficult to move the injured area freely. There is often some bruising, which begins to appear some hours after injury and spreads away from the area. Over time this bruising will change colour as the blood which forms it clots and heals. When assessed by a physiotherapist, the area is swollen and painful, but the bones do not move excessively relative to each other – they remain stable.

• **Grade (III)** injury is a complete rupture of the ligament with some or all of the ligament fibres actually snapping. There is considerable pain with immediate swelling over the whole joint. It is impossible to use the joint and the injury is often painful, even at rest. The joint is unstable when examined, meaning that the bones are not held in place correctly. This is the most severe injury, with recovery time reflecting its severity. It often takes longer to recover from a ligament rupture than from a fracture (broken bone), and in some cases a rupture may need to be surgically repaired.

Muscle strains are again subdivided, this time into four categories with muscle aching and bruising in addition to these (*see* table 3.5, overleaf). Following intense exercise, your muscles are often sore a couple of days afterwards. This is called *delayed onset muscle soreness* (DOMS) and, although common, can actually be classified as a micro-injury. Local

Table 3.5	Muscle injuries
Grading	**What you feel and see**
DOMS[a]	Muscle aching and stiffness 24–48 hours after intense training.
Contusion	Pain and bruising locally with some travelling away from the injury. Tight drum-like muscle, giving slight throbbing at rest.
(i)	Mild strain with local pain and slight stiffness. Pain increases slightly with isometric muscle contraction, but no pain at rest.
(ii)	Moderate strain with more intense pain extending over a greater area. Pain increases substantially with isometric muscle contraction and the muscle may be painful at rest. You can feel a thickened nodule in the muscle.
(iii)	Severe strain with marked bruising and swelling. Pain so intense that you are unwilling to perform an isometric contraction. Pain and throbbing at rest – muscle requires support.
Rupture	Profuse bleeding with severe impairment of function. You cannot contract or stretch the muscle at all. Intense pain even at rest.

[a] Delayed onset muscle soreness

muscle cells are damaged at a microscopic level, causing swelling and pressure which results in the heavy aching familiar to most athletes.

Next in terms of injury intensity is the *contusion*, or muscle bruise. This can occur, for example, in rugby through a heavy tackle or in hockey from being struck by the ball. Some of your smallest blood vessels (capillaries) are damaged, releasing blood which makes up the bruise. Each muscle is surrounded by a thin membrane a little like a cellophane bag. If the bruising is contained by the bag, the swelling stays close to the injury, but if the knock is intense enough to split the muscle membrane, the bruising will spread beyond the injured area. Commonly, this spread of bruising is dragged down by gravity; for example, the bruising from a thigh contusion often extends down to the knee.

Muscle *strains* are graded from one to four (i–iv), covering mild, moderate and severe types,

and finally muscle rupture. Mild strains occur when a few of the muscle fibres are injured. Pain is mild and stays close to the injured area (well localised). Tensing the muscle (isometric contraction) causes a slight ache, which increases if the muscle is tensed harder. A moderate strain is slightly more severe with a larger area of muscle affected. The area feels tense due to internal bleeding within the muscle, and pain is more marked, occurring even when the muscle is lightly contracted. Severe strain sees more profuse bruising and this may burst through the membrane covering the muscle, to spread away from the injured area. Often pain is so severe that you are not able to tense the muscle at all – a process called *pain inhibition*. Finally, a rapidly applied large force may cause the muscle to snap completely, called a *rupture*. You are not able to move the muscle or the limb at all, and bruising is much greater.

Terms you should know:

Exercise progression – increasing the exercise overload to keep pace with tissue change (adaptation).

FITT – mnemonic standing for *Frequency, Intensity, Time,* and *Type.* These variables together make up exercise overload.

Lag phase – period following injury during which tissue is healing but its strength does not increase.

Overload – the challenge placed upon the body during exercise.

Range of motion – how far you are able to move a joint.

Regeneration phase – period of maximum tissue growth and repair following injury.

Remodelling phase – period of healing when new tissue growth is complete and tissue modification begins.

Training intensity – how hard an exercise is (e.g. speed of running or amount of weight lifted).

Training volume – how much exercise is performed (e.g. sets and repetitions, or mileage).

'S' factors – variables making up a fitness programme: stamina, suppleness, strength, spirit, speed, skill and specificity.

SAID – mnemonic standing for *Specific Adaptation to Imposed Demand,* used to describe the process of training specificity.

Specificity – matching an exercise to the precise requirements of a sport or activity.

Supercompensation – the method by which tissue microscopically damaged by exercise is rebuilt to become stronger.

FOOT AND ANKLE

In jumping and running sports, where the ankle area is put under intense pressure, ankle injuries account for over one quarter (25%) of all sports injuries. The foot is your only contact with the ground, and it has to withstand forces which are twice or three times your own bodyweight. Doing this once would be bad enough, but, when running, the foot does this 5000 times in each hour.

ANKLE SPRAIN

The ankle joint is formed between the bottom of the shin bones and the rear foot bones. You actually have two rear foot bones: the *heel*

(calcaneus) and *ankle bone* itself on top (talus) (*see* fig 4.1). The ankle bone sits like a square mortise within the two shin bones. As you point your foot downwards and upwards, the ankle bone slides between the shin bones. It is held in place by two sets of ligaments: on the inside of the ankle is the medial ligament; and on the outside, the lateral ligament. Closer inspection of the lateral ligament shows it to be made up of three bands: the front one pointing forwards, the middle band pointing to the floor and the rear band pointing backwards. When you sprain your ankle, it is the front band of the lateral ligament which is most commonly injured. You can feel this band by placing your

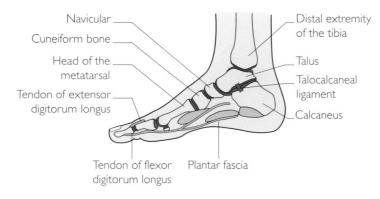

Navicular
Cuneiform bone
Head of the metatarsal
Tendon of extensor digitorum longus
Tendon of flexor digitorum longus
Plantar fascia
Distal extremity of the tibia
Talus
Talocalcaneal ligament
Calcaneus

Figure 4.1 Structure of the ankle

finger on the point of the outer ankle bone and moving your finger forwards and downwards slightly into the hollow part of the joint. Your finger now rests on the front (anterior) band of the ligament.

> **Keypoint**
> With an ankle sprain it is the front (anterior) band of the lateral ankle ligament which is most commonly injured.

Ankle sprain occurs when you go over on the ankle, forcing the sole of your foot inwards. As you are normally moving forwards, either walking or running, when this happens your body continues moving and your foot stays beneath you. The result is that the foot moves inwards and downwards (inversion and plantar flexion), stressing the front of the ligament, rather than the back.

We have seen in chapter 3 that three grades of ligament injury can occur, depending on the intensity of the injury. With a grade (I) ankle sprain there is very little tissue damage. There will be moderate pain with some local swelling which forms gradually after injury and rests on the outside of your ankle between your ankle bone and heel. You will be able to walk on your ankle, but will find it a little painful to turn your body when your foot is fixed on the floor. A grade (II) injury involves damage to more of your ligament fibres, and in some cases a portion of your ligament may detach from the ankle bone. Swelling is far greater and accumulates more quickly, with the whole of the outside of your ankle covered like a puffy balloon. Pain is now intense and it is very difficult to walk without support. There is often some bruising, which begins to appear a few hours after injury and lies beneath your outer ankle bone. When assessed by a physiotherapist, the ankle is swollen and painful, but the bones do not move excessively relative to each other – they remain stable.

Grade (III) injury is a complete rupture of the ligament with some or all of your ligament fibres snapping. There is considerable pain with immediate swelling over the whole of the outer ankle. It is impossible to walk, and extremely painful just to stand. Your ankle is unstable when examined, meaning that the bones are not held in place correctly. Unfortunately, it often takes longer to recover from an ankle ligament rupture than from an ankle fracture, and in some cases a rupture of this type may need to be surgically repaired.

> **Keypoint**
> It can take longer to recover from a severe ankle ligament injury than from an ankle bone break (fracture).

Treatment aims initially are to reduce pain and swelling and facilitate tissue healing. Later the area must be re-strengthened and walking and running gait re-educated to avoid limping.

TAPING

An acute ankle sprain may be supported by an ankle immobiliser (rigid cast) (*see* fig 2.1b, page 11), a brace or taping. An ankle immobiliser

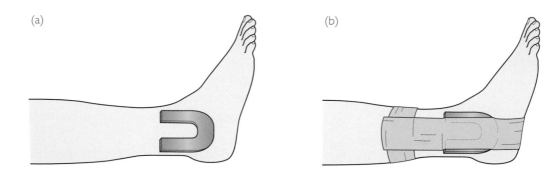

(a)   (b)

Figure 4.2 Ankle lock taping: (a) a half-moon-shaped piece of foam is placed below the ankle bone (b) tape stirrups run over the pad

protects the joint against all ankle movement, while a brace protects against inward and outward movement but allows up and down actions. Taping may be tailored to the precise requirements of your injury. Sprain to the outside of the joint is supported using an ankle lock taping (*see* fig 4.2).

Begin by checking that you don't have any cuts or abrasions on the skin and that the skin is clean. If the skin is cut or delicate, apply a foam underwrap.

- A half-moon-shaped piece of felt or foam is placed below the outer ankle bone (lateral malleolus), to prevent swelling concentrating here to form a pocket of fluid (*see* fig 4.2a).

- An anchor is placed around the upper shin, being cautious not to pull this tightly which may restrict the blood flowing through the calf.

- Two U-shaped taping stirrups are placed beneath the ankle, running from the inside of the shin under the heel bone to the outside. Pulling the tape in this outward direction

causes the ankle and heel to swing outwards (eversion) to shorten and protect the ligament.

- The stirrups attach to the anchors, giving a firmer hold and ensuring that the tape does not slip (*see* fig 4.2b).

- The ankle lock can be finished using adherent taping which sticks to itself rather than to the skin. This is applied in a figure-of-eight. Begin on the outside of the foot just back from the little toe (mid-foot area), and wrap the tape across the top of the foot, and then around beneath the sole.

- As the tape emerges by the little toe again, take the second layer up across the front of the ankle to the outside, pulling on the tape to provide tension which draws the foot upwards (dorsiflexion) and outwards (eversion) to shorten the outer ankle ligament.

- This layer of tape passes around the back of the Achilles and then over onto the front of the

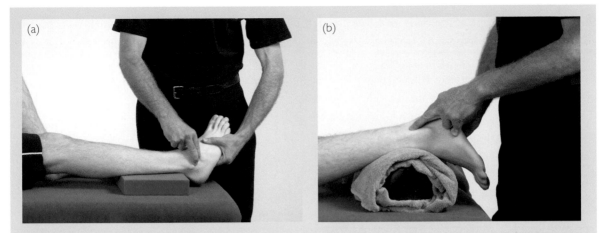

Figure 4.3 Ankle massage: (a) specific massage along Achilles (b) deep transverse friction (DTF) massage

ankle and inside of the foot overlapping the first layer of tape by half its width. Tension on the tape is quite strong over the foot and ankle but reduces as the tape progresses up the shin.

When the tape is on, check that it does not restrict the circulation. Compress the nail of the big toe between your thumb and forefinger until the nail bed (flesh beneath the toe) goes white. Release the pressure and check that the normal pink colour of the skin returns within 15–30 seconds. If it does not, blood is not getting through to the toes because the tape is too tight. Take the tape off and rest for 15 minutes before reapplying the tape under less tension.

MASSAGE

As pain subsides and we move into the sub-acute phase of the injury (3–4 days after injury), gentle massage may be used to ease swelling and enhance circulation. Two types of massage are used: *general* and *specific*. General massage is used over the whole of the lower leg, while specific massage is used over the outer ankle. Ankle swelling can be relieved using effleurage movements.

> ### Keypoint
> *General* massage is used over a whole limb or number of body parts, while *specific* massage addresses a single structure.

Ask the injured person to lie down with their legs stretched out. Place a cushion or folded towel beneath their knees for comfort. Begin with general massage at the foot and contour your hands around the ankle and calf. The pressure should be on the upward stroke, moving swelling from the ankle to the knee. Release the pressure and glide your hands back to the foot. Perform five strokes like this on the centre of the ankle and shin, five on the outside and five on the inside. Next, use your fingertips (keeping the fingers together) and press them into the sides of the ankle between the ankle bone and Achilles as you stroke upwards. Again, perform five strokes like this. Moving to specific massage, use your thumbs or first and middle fingers together (*see* fig 4.3a, page 43) to perform small circles around the outer ankle bone. Begin with light pressure and increase this gradually as the swelling eases. Finish the massage session with the general massage strokes again.

Later in the healing process swelling will have stopped forming and the problem comes not from fresh swelling as a watery fluid, but from congealed swelling which has stuck to the tissues in the local area becoming initially gel-like and eventually fibrous. This can be managed using deep transverse friction (DTF) massage (*see* fig 4.3b, page 43). Again you should use the first and middle fingers together as a single tool. This time, however, rather than moving across the skin, you should press into the skin directly over the healing ligament. Maintain this pressure and move your fingers to and fro so that the skin and fingers move as a single unit. This imparts the force of the friction massage to the tissue beneath the skin rather than to the skin itself. To increase the effectiveness of DTF, tighten the ligament by drawing the foot down and in (plantar flexion and inversion) and maintain this position throughout the DTF treatment. It is common for your foot to feel slightly tender with this treatment, but if it is very painful, stop.

EXERCISES

Remember that initially you should not exercise where the injury is severe (grade (II) or (III) sprain). Once pain begins to subside and healing has begun you can start gentle exercise from 3 or 4 days after injury. Begin using non-weight bearing exercise, that is sitting or lying with your foot off the ground. When movement starts to ease, exercise is progressed to partial weight bearing positions and resistance training.

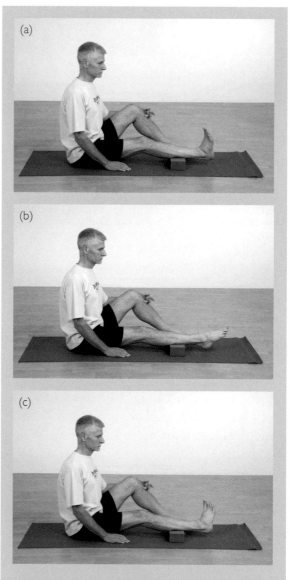

Figure 4.4 Ankle mobilising: (a) dorsiflexion (b) plantarflexion (c) inversion and eversion

Definition

Non-weight bearing exercise is performed taking no weight through a limb. Partial weight bearing exercise takes some weight, and full weight bearing takes all of your bodyweight through a limb.

Ankle mobilising

Purpose

To stimulate local circulation and begin to reduce swelling.

Preparation

Sit on the floor with your legs out straight in front of you. Place a block, cushion or rolled towel under your calf.

Action

There are three components to this exercise. First, pull your toes and foot up and down (dorsiflexion and plantar flexion). Second, pull them inwards and outwards (inversion and eversion). Third, circle your whole foot, keeping the shin bone fixed (circumduction) (*see* fig 4.4, page 44).

Tips

Begin by doing these exercises gently and rhythmically, easing into the painful and stiff areas of movement, but not forcing. As stiffness reduces, press a little harder at the ends of each movement to try to stretch the tissues.

As pain eases you should begin simple walking drills. When walking forwards make sure you keep your feet parallel rather than turning the injured foot out. Often the upward movement of your foot (dorsiflexion) is tight due to swelling, and there is a tendency to turn the foot outwards to relieve the pressure on the joint. Rather than doing this, which will cause you to limp, shorten the distance between each step and slow down your pace, using your walking as a rehab drill. Next, practise backward walking, again ensuring that your feet stay parallel to each other. When you can do both forwards and backwards walking confidently, start sideways walking and zigzag walking. These will be harder and may be slightly uncomfortable to begin because your ankle will move differently. Start slowly and build up to a marching pace.

Resistance training can be performed using a cushion or gym ball to begin.

Isometric ankle strengthening

Purpose

To strengthen the muscles which support your outer ankle (evertor muscles).

Preparation

Sit on the floor, side on to a wall with a gym ball or cushion sandwiched between your outer ankle and the wall (*see* fig 4.5, page 46).

Action

Keep you shin still (kneecap facing the ceiling) and press your foot outwards and into the ball/cushion (ankle eversion). Hold the end position tight for 5–10 seconds and then release, performing 2 or 3 sets of 5–8 reps.

Tips

Using a *gym ball* provides a greater resistance as it is springier than a cushion. A similar resistance

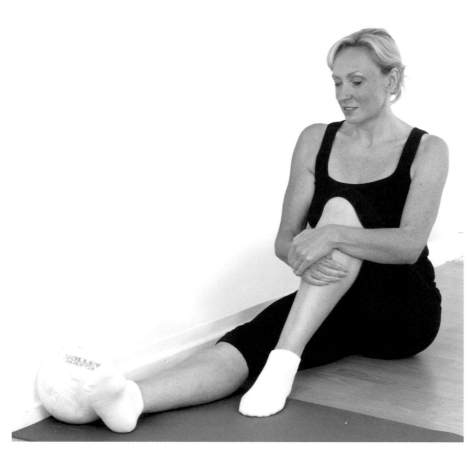

Figure 4.5 Isometric ankle strengthening

can be created using a *resistance band*. Loop the band around your ankle and tie it to a piece of furniture on the inside of your ankle. Again, keep your shin still and turn your ankle out, holding the end position to tighten the muscles.

Two stretching exercises are important. The first encourages upward bending of the ankle (dorsiflexion) to improve walking, while the second stretches the ligament itself by combining downward and inward movement (plantar flexion and inversion).

Ankle bending
Purpose
To improve the upwards bending action of the ankle.

Preparation
Place your injured foot on a chair and keep your foot flat throughout the exercise (do not allow your heal to lift).

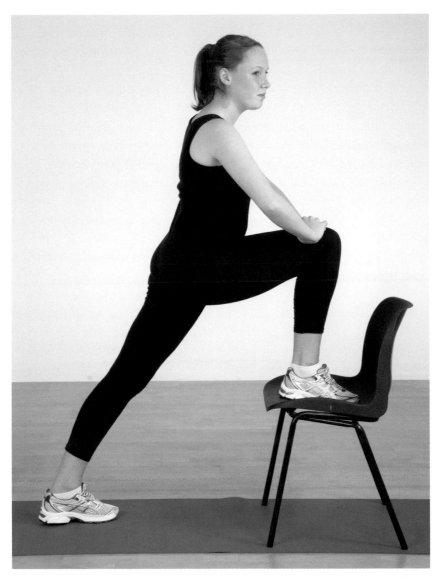

Figure 4.6 Ankle bending

Action

Press your knee forwards towards the chair back (*see* fig 4.6). Release the stretch and then press forwards again, this time aiming your kneecap inwards. Release again and finally lunge, aiming your kneecap outwards. These three movements form the parts of a single exercise, and you should perform three exercises in total.

Tips

By aiming the kneecap forwards, forwards and inwards, and then forwards and outwards, you place pressure on different parts of your ankle joint to ensure a comprehensive stretch. You should use two timings, each at different training sessions. First, hold the forward pressure for 5–15 seconds, performing 3 reps, and in the next session use a pulsing action, gently pressing and releasing rhythmically 10 times in each forward position.

Outer ankle stretch

Purpose

To stretch the outer ligament directly.

Preparation

Sit forwards on a chair and cross your injured leg (*see* fig 4.7, page 49). Fix your injured ankle with one hand and then reach underneath your foot with your opposite hand.

Action

Gently draw your foot downwards and inwards, keeping your shin fixed. Hold the stretched position for 5–15 seconds and then release. Perform 3 reps daily.

Tips

Altering the foot position will vary the part of the ligament that receives the stretch.

You now need to progress your exercise from slow controlled strength work and stretching to faster power-based actions. You actually began this with the walking drills described above, and the first step is to speed up these drills to a vigorous marching pace and then to slow running. Begin by using a scout pace, walking briskly for 20 steps and then jogging for 20 steps. Do this for each of the directions (forwards, backwards, sideways), making sure that your path is clear and flat, avoiding any uneven ground that could trip you. When confident with a jogging pace, progress once again, this time to jumping drills, first on both legs and then on the single leg. Again, the direction also progresses, forwards/backwards being easier than sideways, which is itself easier than twisting and jumping.

To create a greater variety of movements and to improve your ankle balance sense (proprioception), you will need to practise standing on an uneven surface. This could be, for example, a foam cushion from the sofa or a specially designed wobble board. Begin standing on one leg on a flat surface, when you are confident to move onto an uneven surface.

Ankle balance

Purpose

To improve ankle balance sense and stability.

Preparation

Place a flat cushion (sofa cushion) or towel on the floor, close to a wall for support should you need it.

Action

Stand on your injured leg, bending your uninjured leg at the knee (*see* fig 4.8, page 50). Initially, try to keep your balance for 30–60 seconds. As your ankle balance sense begins to improve, progress the exercise by performing small squats (quarter squats) on the floor and then turning the body from side to side. Build up the amount of time you spend on the board from 1–2 minutes to 5–6 minutes twice daily.

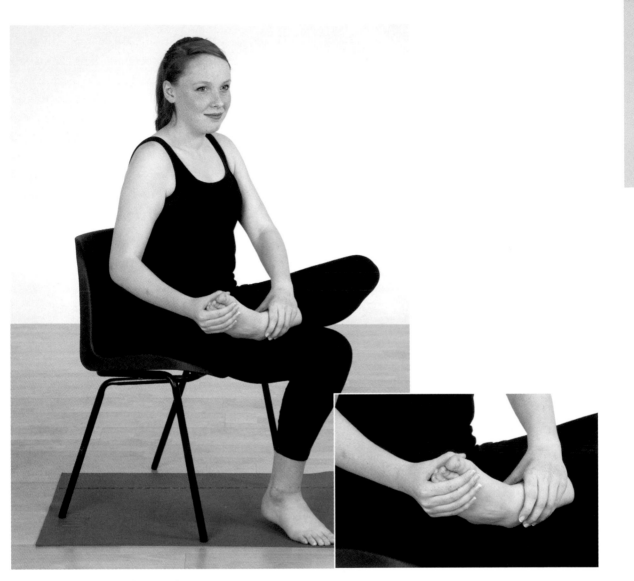

Figure 4.7 Outer ankle stretch

Tips

You will find that you wobble and all of the muscles around your ankle work hard to protect your ankle and keep it stable.

BIG TOE JOINT

Your big toe joint or ball of the foot can suffer from a variety of sports-related conditions. Like other joints, it is moved by muscles and supported by ligament. However, uniquely it also has two small additional bones underneath it called

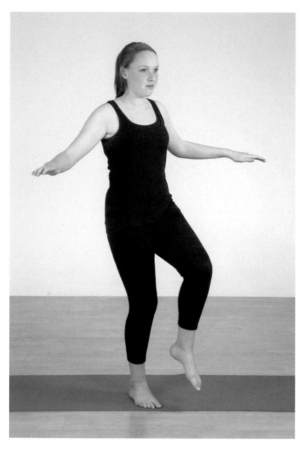

Figure 4.8 Ankle balance exercise

The second condition, which is common, is wear and tear of the big toe joint. This begins as a mild swelling and roughening of the joint, which can progress to stiffness and angling inwards of the joint – conditions called *Hallux rigidus* and *Hallux valus*, respectively. Where angulation of the joint occurs, the outer knuckle of the toe may press against the inside of the shoe, creating a thickened area or bunion. This can be relieved using a gel pad, making walking and running activities considerably more comfortable. The hard skin should be removed professionally by a registered chiropodist. In all of these conditions, treatment is required in the acute phase of injury and rehabilitation as the joint recovers.

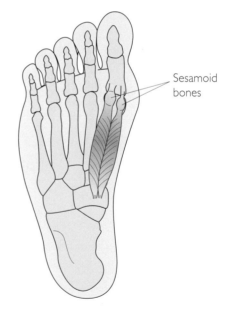

Sesamoid bones

Figure 4.9 The big toe joint

sesamoids (*see* fig 4.9), and a flat plate supporting its undersurface that acts as the connecting junction for muscles and ligaments. This complex structure reflects an important function of the joint, which is to provide the push off in walking and running, where this relatively small joint takes most of your bodyweight. The structures beneath the joint can be torn in a condition called *turf toe*. This occurs if the toe is forced to bend too far (*see* fig 4.10), especially if a player falls onto you, forcing the toes upwards.

TAPING

The big toe joint is taped using strips of non-elastic tape secured to tape anchors placed around the forefoot and toe (*see* fig 4.11). The aim is to limit the upward bending of the joint and give the area a chance to recover. Wearing a stiffer-soled shoe will also help to restrict movement.

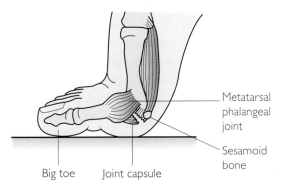

Big toe   Joint capsule

Metatarsal phalangeal joint

Sesamoid bone

Figure 4.10 Turf toe injury

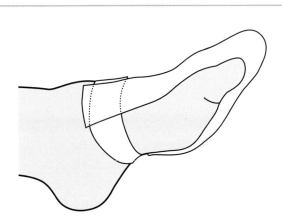

Figure 4.11 Big toe taping: tape anchors travel from the stirrup over the big toe

JOINT MOBILISATION

When the joint is very stiff, but not inflamed, joint mobilisation is helpful. Here, you try to move the joint not by forcing the stiff upward and downward movements of the joint, but instead by focusing on the *joint play*. Joint play (accessory movement) is the springy feeling of a healthy joint, which is normally lost first, before you notice your toe becoming stiff. In a healthy joint, movement should be free, but more importantly the joint should feel elastic and not brittle. Contrast how a child's joints feel compared to an adult's. The child is more flexible, but also their joints feel more elastic – the elasticity is because they have more joint play. While we inevitably lose some joint play as we get older, it is possible to both slow this process down and reverse it slightly. For example, many individuals who regularly practise yoga maintain flexibility and elasticity in their joints into older age.

> **Keypoint**
> *Accessory movement* or *joint play* gives a joint its healthy springy feeling. This is lost following injury and must be regained with joint mobilisation.

To improve joint play in the big toe joint you need to pull (traction) the joint gently (*see* fig 4.12, overleaf). The action is very gentle and rhythmical without any jolting or jarring. Begin by gripping your foot with one hand and your big toe with the other. Gently pull your hands apart in a rhythmical oscillation 20–30 times, aiming to move your hands only millimetres. Initially, you will not be able to feel any movement, but gradually you will find you detect a little creaking in the joint as stiffness begins to ease. If you find it difficult to reach down to your toes, an alternative is to stand and place the heel of you uninjured foot on top of your injured toe. Your action now is to try to drag

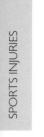

bath or shower, when your tissues are more elastic and your muscles relaxed.

SOLE OF THE FOOT

The sole of the foot can often give severe pain during sport with a condition called *plantar fasciitis*. This affects the tissue supporting the foot arch, which starts to change (maladaption), becoming stiffer and less forgiving. The condition used to be thought to be inflammation, but modern research has shown that in fact, rather than being inflamed, the tissue actually heals incorrectly. The cause is thought to be a combination of footwear and injury. We tend to think of the foot as being quite passive. It sits in the shoe and simply hits the ground with each step as we walk. In the wild, however, the foot is as active as any other part of your body. It moves constantly as we walk, adapting to changes in the terrain. The arch is supported by muscles as well as the plantar fascia, and these muscles should be thick and strong. By wearing shoes, the arch muscles weaken meaning that all of your weight has to be taken by the plantar fascia. This is increased if you are overweight and if you spend a lot of time standing in one place. The arch drops slightly as the plantar fascia is overstretched and it tries to compensate and become stronger by thickening and becoming leathery. Treatment has to address two problems here: the injury to the tissues (pathology) and the change in the body which caused them (dysfunction). You do this by supporting the foot arch until pain begins to ease and then strengthening the foot arch muscles so they can take stress away from the plantar fascia.

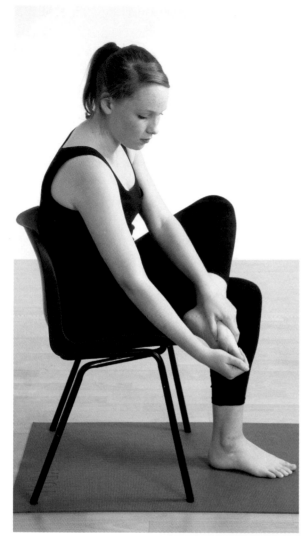

Figure 4.12 Pulling the big toe joint to improve joint play

your foot on the injured leg backwards (towards your heel) using the same gentle oscillation. Use this mobilisation action once a day after a warm

TAPING AND SUPPORT

Plantar fascia taping stretches the length of the sole of the foot from the heel to behind the toes.

- Using non-elastic tape begin with anchors behind the toes and around the heel (*see* fig 4.13a).

- Between these, place strips of tape keeping the foot relaxed and in mid position (don't point the toes) (*see* fig 4.13b). When you stand up you should feel that the arch of your foot is supported, but you are able to move your toes freely.

Another method of supporting your foot arch and resting the plantar fascia is to use an orthotic. This is a shoe insert which has a shaped cup for your heel and a dome to support your arch. In addition, an *orthotic* will keep your heel bone aligned, stopping you from turning your heel in and rolling over on the inner edge of your shoe.

Pain may often be relieved by using pressure into the sole of the foot using massage. This may

Definition

An *orthotic* is a shoe insert designed to alter motion of the foot. It often has a dome to support the foot arch and a cup shaped to the heel. Small blocks (posts) are placed beneath the orthotic to alter contact between the foot and the ground.

be performed by a physiotherapist using a pressure massage tool (*see* fig 4.14, overleaf) and at home by gently pressing your foot down onto a golf ball and moving your foot in a circular motion to create a similar massaging effect.

EXERCISES

Your foot pain may be relieved by slowly stretching the plantar fascia. As pain eases, it is time to strengthen the muscles of your foot to get them to support your arch. Strong foot muscles take over the job done by taping and an orthotic.

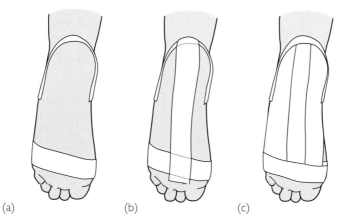

(a)   (b)   (c)

Figure 4.13 Sole of foot (plantarfascia) taping: (a) stirrups are placed around the forefoot and heel (b) several stirrups are combined to add strength (c) completed taping

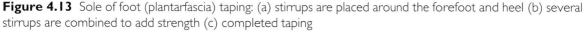

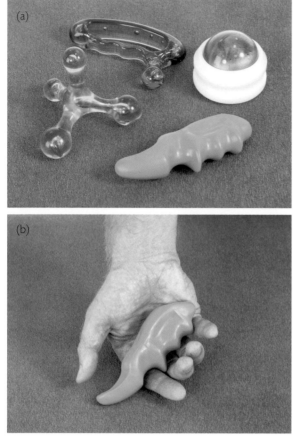

Figure 4.14 A selection of pressure massage tools

Plantar fascia stretching

Purpose
To lengthen the plantar fascia and ease pain.

Preparation
Begin in bare feet close to a wall with your injured foot forwards (*see* fig 4.15a, page 55).

Action
Place your big toe flat against the wall, keeping the sole of your foot on the floor. Your big toe joint should be bent to 90 degrees or thereabouts.

Initially, this stretch may be sufficient. If pain permits, slowly press your knee forwards towards the wall so that your ankle bends (*see* fig 4.15b, page 55). Hold the stretched position for 5–10 seconds initially, building up to 20–30 seconds after a few days. Practise the exercise twice daily for 1 or 2 reps only.

Tips
It often takes a little shuffling to get into this position. Bend you big toe joint only as far as is comfortable. If the joint is stiff, you may bend it less but still get an adequate plantar fascia stretch by pressing your knee closer to the wall.

Arch lift – sitting

Purpose
To begin strengthening the foot arch muscles.

Preparation
Begin sitting with your bare foot flat on the floor and shin bone vertical.

Action
Take your leg weight onto the inner aspect of your foot and allow the arch to flatten, and then take the weight over the outer aspect and increase the arch of your foot. As you increase the arch height, imagine that you are drawing the ball of your foot towards your heel (*see* fig 4.16, page 55).

Tips
Do not scrunch up your toes (toe flexion), but pull with the ball of your foot instead. As you increase your arch height, your training partner should still be able to lift your toes (toe extension), showing that you are using your arch muscles and not your toe-bending muscles.

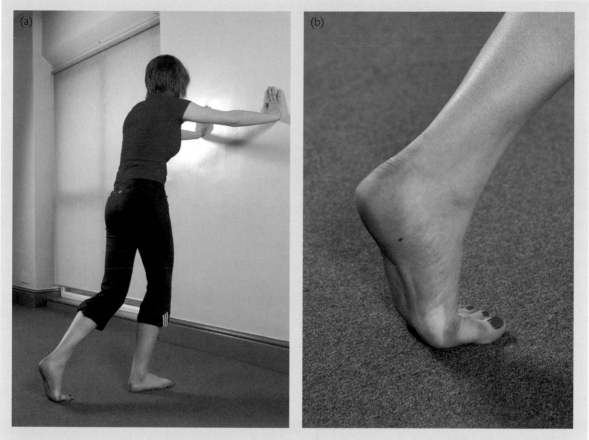

Figure 4.15 Plantar fascia stretching: (a) body position – leaning against the wall (b) big toe joint action

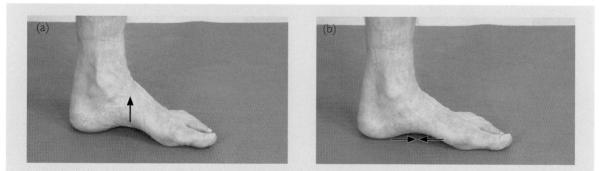

Figure 4.16 Arch lift – sitting: (a) lift the arch (b) draw the ball of the foot towards the heel

Arch lift and lunge

Purpose

To progress foot arch strength.

Preparation

Begin kneeling on a non-carpeted floor in bare feet. Step forwards into a lunge position with your right foot.

Action

Initially, take your weight onto your back (right) foot. Increase the height of your foot arch by taking weight over the outside of your foot and moving your knee over the foot outer edge. Hold the high arch position and bring your bodyweight forwards, pressing onto the front foot while maintaining the high arch position (see fig 4.17).

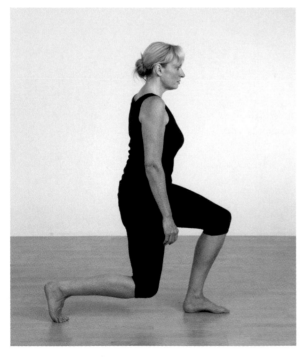

Figure 4.17 Arch lift and lunge

Tips

The knee movement in this exercise is quite subtle. It can help to draw a vertical line on the centre of your kneecap and a line from your 4th toe towards your ankle. As you press your knee forwards, try to line up the knee and foot lines. To take less weight on the foot the exercise may be performed with the knee on the ground.

TOENAIL AND SKIN PROBLEMS

Black toe, or *runners nail*, is a condition where blood builds up beneath the toenail (subungual haematoma). Direct pressure on the toenail is the normal cause, either from tight fitting training shoes when running downhill or from someone stepping on the foot. Pressure builds up in the space between the nail and the delicate flesh beneath (nail bed), causing pain and throbbing. If sufficient blood is released the pressure may be so great that the nail actually lifts away from the nail bed. When the condition is caught soon enough the bruise may be released by a therapist puncturing the nail with a sterile needle. A special device is available for this job, called a *nail trephine*, which uses sterile disposable flat needles.

> **Definition**
> A *nail trephine* is a disposable needle device used for sterile puncture of a nail to release underlying blood from a runner's 'black toe'.

Nail bed infection and *ingrown nail* may occur especially in the big toe. These are often a result of cutting the toenails too short, which uncovers the delicate skin to the side of the nail. If small nail splinters are caused when the nails are cut, these may press into the delicate toe flesh when shoes are too tight. Treatment is to see a chiropodist immediately as the ingrown nail may be treated (painlessly) and an antibiotic cream given for the infection.

Blisters often occur as a result of direct squeezing (compression) or rubbing (shearing) forces on the skin. If the front part (toe box) of a running shoe is too tight, blisters may form over the little toe, and if the big toe touches the 2nd toe, blisters can be formed between the two toes. When recently formed, blisters may be drained through a puncture hole by a therapist. A sterile needle held parallel to the skin is used to puncture the side of the blister. This technique leaves a flap of skin to protect the area, and a sterile dressing is applied to the foot to stop infection.

Athlete's foot (tinea pedis) is a fungal infection which affects the skin of the feet, and the same fungus is the cause of jock itch (tinea cruis). Athlete's foot occurs between the toes where moisture and warmth build up. This is unfortunately an ideal environment for the fungus to grow; the fungus is then commonly transmitted throughout communal changing areas. The skin becomes white, itchy and scaly and has a characteristic smell. Therapists normally remove the scaled skin with surgical spirit and then apply an antifungal powder or cream. Tea tree oil cream can be an effective home treatment, and socks should be changed regularly. Avoid sharing towels and do not go barefoot in communal changing rooms until the condition has cleared. Persistent cases should be referred to a chiropodist.

Terms you should know:

Accessory movement (joint play) — the springy feeling of a healthy joint.

Ankle lock — taping used to support a sprain to the outside of the ankle joint.

DTF — deep transverse friction massage.

Hallux — anatomical term for the big toe.

Ingrown nail — toenail growing into the flesh beneath it (nail bed). Technically called *onychocryptosis*.

Lateral ligament — outer ankle ligament made up of three bands.

Maladaption — change for the worse as a result of stress imposed on tissue.

Non-weight bearing — keeping the foot off the ground so that no bodyweight is taken through the lower limb joints.

Orthotic — shoe insert designed to correct foot motion.

Proprioception — joint balance sense.

Sesamoid — an extra (accessory) bone embedded within a tendon.

Toe box — front part of a running shoe that covers the toes.

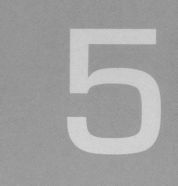

// CALF AND SHIN

Calf and shin injuries fall broadly into two categories. Injuries which occur suddenly (trauma) typically affect the calf muscle, while injuries which occur slowly (overuse) are typically seen in the shin muscle. The Achilles can suffer from both types, with pain coming on gradually called *tendinopathy*, and that coming on suddenly *tendon rupture*.

CALF TEAR

The calf actually consists of a long and a short calf muscle. They both work over the ankle, but the long one goes above the knee (gastrocnemius) and the short one below (soleus). This fact is important when stretching, because the long calf muscle is more effectively stretched with the knee locked out straight and the short muscle with the knee allowed to bend.

> **Keypoint**
> The calf has both a long muscle attaching above the knee and a short muscle attaching below. To stretch both, exercises must be performed with the knee straight and then with the knee bent.

In addition, the long calf muscle more commonly tears with explosive actions such as lunging for a ball in tennis; in fact, a tear of this muscle was once traditionally called *tennis leg*. The long calf muscle consists of two portions, or *bellies*, and normally one is injured rather than both. You may have been running and slipped on some gravel, or stepped off a curve awkwardly. You suddenly feel a deep pain in the calf as though someone has kicked you, and it is difficult to walk normally.

TAPING

Initially, it is important to rest the injured muscle to prevent further tissue damage. Unfortunately, our day-to-day jobs often prevent us from resting as we would wish. To protect the calf you should tape the injured muscle. The calf is taped with the heel lifted slightly to relax the injured muscle. Begin with your partner lying on their front. Their shin should rest on a folded towel, with their toes over the end of a bed or bench.

- Begin by placing an anchor of non-elastic adhesive tape around the sole of the foot (*see* fig 5.1a, page 59).

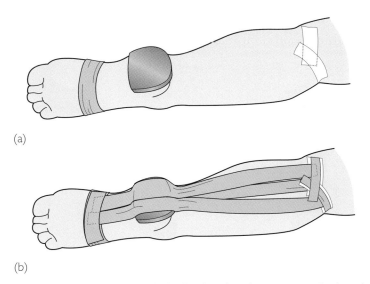

(a)

(b)

Figure 5.1 Calf taping: (a) a pad is placed beneath the heel and anchors are attached to the upper calf (b) reins link anchors

- Next place two anchors at the top of the calf just below the knee, in an upturned 'V' shape. If the shin is very hairy you will need to clip it using scissors or a hair clipper. Do not wet shave the skin as the tape adhesive can irritate the skin afterwards. Clippers take the hair off but leave enough stubble to protect the skin, whereas wet shaping removes the surface layer of skin, exposing the more delicate areas underneath.

- Place a pad made from one or two layers of adhesive felt beneath the heel (*see* fig 5.1a).

- Apply lengths of tape from the foot anchor across the heel to the calf anchors. Two or three may be used depending on the size of the calf muscles (*see* fig 5.1b).

- When the taping has been applied your partner should be able to put their heel on the ground with the heel slightly elevated on the felt pads. The taping is too tight if they have to walk on their toes.

Where the calf injury is very mild (grade I) the full taping may not be required, and local compression can be used instead. You can use simple elasticated tubular bandage or apply local compression and support using strips of adhesive elastic tape. This is applied pre-stretched directly onto the skin and as it recoils it compresses and supports the area.

MASSAGE

General calf massage is performed with your partner lying on their front and their foot supported on a pillow or cushion. Use deep stroking actions from the heel to the calf, and then grip the muscle and lift it slightly away from the

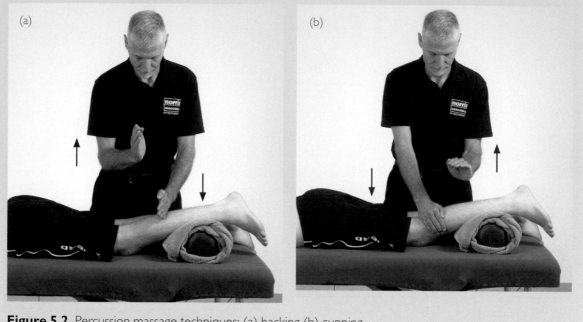

Figure 5.2 Percussion massage techniques: (a) hacking (b) cupping

bone to stretch the tissue widthways. Percussion techniques are used to stimulate the local circulation and may be performed with your fingertips gripped together or using the sides of your hands with your fingers open to soften the hand strike (*see* fig 5.2).

Deeper massage may be given with your partner sitting and their knee bent. Hook your hands around the back of their calf and lean backwards slightly to create deep pressure into the muscle. You can localise the massage using your fingertips or make the pressure more general using the whole of your hand. Deep transverse friction massage (DTF) may also be applied across the muscle fibres which is in the direction of the shin bone.

Ice massage is a useful technique to relieve local pain and increase blood flow. Rather than holding an ice cube it is simpler to fill a polystyrene cup with water and freeze it. When frozen, peel off the rim of the cup to expose the ice (alternatively use an ice-up massager (*see* fig 5.3)). If using ice, put oil on the skin to protect it, and move the ice in small circles over the painful muscle area for 10–15 minutes. The area will be red and numb at the end of the treatment, allowing deep massage to be used or stretching to be performed. The technique is used in the chronic stages of an injury where scar tissue has formed. The scar tissue may be stretched and mobilised using massage in the period after ice application.

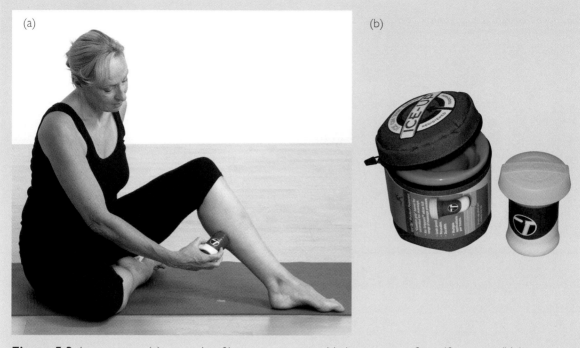

Figure 5.3 Ice massage: (a) example of how to use a portable ice massager for calf massage (b) ice-up massager

Keypoint

Ice massage is used to increase blood flow and ease pain. Use it prior to stretching or mobilising scar tissue in the chronic stage of an injury.

Where you have a tight painful nodule (trigger point) in the muscle, self-massage given using a foam roll or spiky ball can be effective. Sit on the floor with the roll beneath your calf. Allow the weight of your leg to press your calf against the roll. Draw your leg up and down over the roll, allowing your knee to bend and straighten slightly as you do so. For a more intense stimulus to the skin, substitute a spiky ball for the foam roll (*see* fig 5.4, overleaf). Roll your leg up and down and side to side, focusing on the painful area. Initially, your pain may increase slightly as you hit the spot, but it should then quickly subside. Use this self-massage for 2–3 minutes and slowly stretch the calf out afterwards.

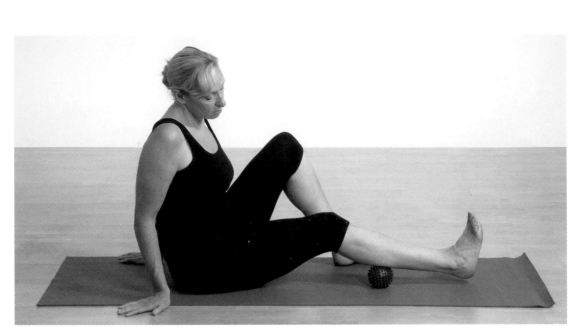

Figure 5.4 Self-massage (calf) with a spiky ball

EXERCISES

Calf stretch

Purpose

To stretch the calf muscles and elongate the healing tissue.

Preparation

Begin leaning up against a wall in a lunge position with your injured leg back, toes on the floor and heel raised.

Action

Lock your knee out straight and press your heel to the ground. Ease into the movement, gently working the heel towards the floor (*see* fig 5.5). Hold the end stretch for 20–30 seconds without bouncing.

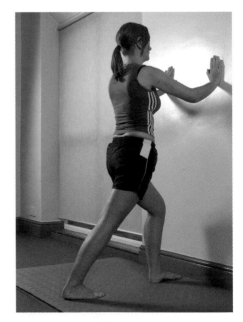

Figure 5.5 Calf stretch

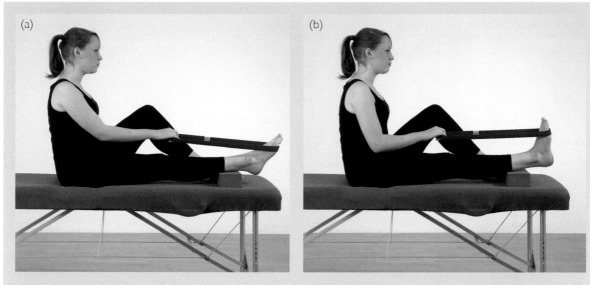

Figure 5.6 Calf tensing using a band: (a) start position (b) using the band, draw your ankle towards you

Tips

The further away from the wall the foot is the greater the angle at the ankle and so the more intense the calf stretch.

Calf tensing using a band

Purpose

To contract and stretch the calf muscle, creating a rhythmical pumping action on the muscle circulation.

Preparation

Begin sitting with your legs straight out in front of you. Hook an exercise band over the ball of your foot (*see* fig 5.6a).

Action

Keeping your leg straight, flex your ankle to point your toes away from you (plantar flexion). Pause in this position and then allow the band to draw your ankle back towards you (dorsiflexion) (*see* fig 5.6b). Perform 10 reps of this movement in a smooth controlled manner.

Tips

To emphasise the stretching aspect of this exercise, point the toes for a count of 2 and relax the foot allowing the band to stretch the calf for a count of 4.

Heel raise

Purpose

To strengthen the calf muscles.

Preparation

Begin facing a wall or back of a chair with your toes resting on a block or thick book. Ensure that your heels are on the floor.

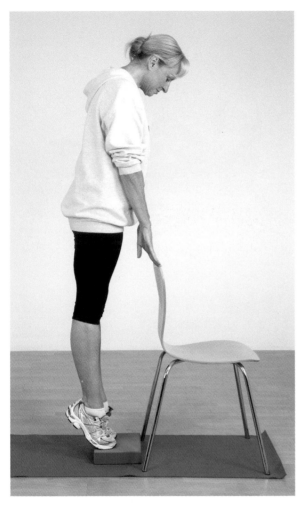

Figure 5.7 Heel raise

exercise as it angles the shin and takes some of the stretch from the calf. If your calf feels tight or painful, use a lower block. Alternatively, if the calf is very weak, raise the body using both legs and lower using just the injured one.

Sprint start

Purpose

To build the power and speed of the calf muscles.

Preparation

Begin on the balls of your feet in a sprint start position with your hips high, arms straight and legs at an angle of 45 degrees to the floor.

Action

Begin by alternatively lifting your heels and pressing them down onto the floor for 5 reps each leg, allowing your knees to bend naturally. Next, keep your right leg straight and bend your left knee. Now, use your right calf muscle power to push your toes into the floor and rock your hips forwards for 5 reps, keeping the toes on the floor. Finally, press your right toes into the floor and take a pace forwards with your right leg as though beginning a race (*see* fig 5.8, page 65). Repeat with the left leg.

Tips

The exercise becomes more demanding when you take less weight on your arms and more on your feet.

Hop and hold

Purpose

To perform final calf strengthening prior to sports competition.

Action

Keeping your leg straight and body aligned, raise up onto your toes. Pause in the upper position and then lower under control (see fig 5.7).

Tips

There is a tendency to allow your hips to fall backwards (sticking your bottom out) with this

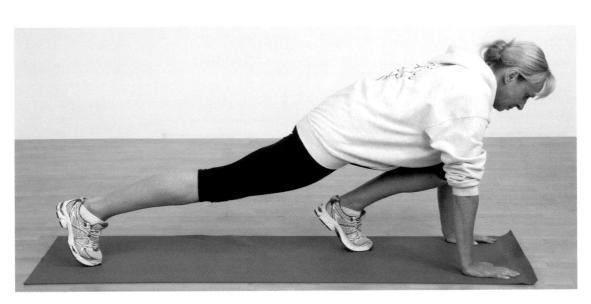

Figure 5.8 Sprint start

Preparation

Mark a cross on the floor with two pieces of tape each about ½ metre long. Begin the exercise by warming up the calf using fast walking on the spot and then gentle jogging for a total of 5 minutes until sweating slightly.

Action

Hop forwards and backwards for 10 reps over the centre of the cross, making each step about 20 cm long initially. Pause and then hop side to side for the same distance. Progress the exercise by hopping higher and holding the landing position for 1–2 seconds. Finally combine the two actions by hopping high forwards, backwards and side to side, holding each landing position for 1–2 seconds.

Tips

By holding the exercise the calf stretch is emphasised. Using a continuous action places less focus on the stretch but builds up the bouncing (ballistic) nature of the muscle contraction. Use both techniques for variety.

ACHILLES TENDON

The Achilles is the largest tendon in the body measuring on average about 15 cm in length and 2 cm in thickness. It is extremely strong with laboratory experiments showing that it is capable of withstanding loads of up to 17 times the bodyweight.

Keypoint

The Achilles is the largest tendon in the body. It is capable of withstanding loads of up to 17 times your bodyweight.

The Achilles joins the two large calf muscles (gastrocnemius and soleus) to the heel bone (calcaneus) and transmits the power of the calf into the foot to allow you to push off against the ground during walking and running. The tendon passes across the back of the heel bone, where it is separated from the bone by a balloon-like structure, the *Achilles bursa*. The Achilles is highly elastic, a function which is increased by the fact that the tendon twists through 90 degrees throughout its length, and unwinds as it is stretched. Each end of the tendon has a good blood supply, but in the central portion the blood flow it not as good. If the tendon snaps (ruptures) it is often this portion which is affected.

Two injuries are seen in sport: *Achilles tendinopathy*, which involves pain, swelling and thickening along the tendon; and *tendon rupture*. Tendinopathy normally begins as a dull tendon ache after running. As the condition progresses there is even pain at rest. The tendon appears swollen and thicker than the other side. You often find the tendon gets stiff after sitting for long periods, and it is stiff and painful first thing in the morning. It often takes 10–12 steps of 'hobbling' on your toes before you are able to actually get your heel down to the ground. When we look at the tendon under a microscope we see that rather than being inflamed, the nature of the tendon tissue and cells within it have actually changed and new blood vessels have grown into the area. In short the tendon has responded to excessive stress by incorrect healing. This altered healing response holds the key to treatment. Rest is only required while pain is intense; too much rest will not help this condition. The tendon needs to be physically stressed to encourage the healing response to get back on track.

Definition

The *Achilles tendon* is the tendon that attaches the calf muscles to the heel bone.

REST AND TAPING

You must rest from the activity which is causing you pain. Although this injury eventually responds well to controlled loading, it will get worse if not rested initially from high impact forces.

The taping that we used for a calf tear (*see* fig 5.1, page 59) may also be used for the Achilles tendon. In cases where pain is less acute a simple heel raise may be all that is required to take the stretch off the tendon. Ladies often find wearing a higher-heeled shoe helps. Ice may be used to reduce pain, but an ice water soak is better than the direct application of ice as the tendon is thin and susceptible to ice burns.

As pain eases, stretching and tendon loading are required. These will both ease pain, so can be begun before your tendon is completely pain free.

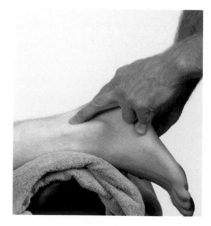

Figure 5.9 Achilles specific massage

MASSAGE

Massage to the Achilles is a very effective way of relieving pain and a useful technique to prepare the tendon for exercise. Begin with your partner lying on their front with their shin supported on a folded towel, tendon relaxed. Massage along the edges of the tendon with your fingertips using small circular movements. Focus on the tendon itself and the area between the base of the tendon and the foot (Kager triangle). Begin quite superficially and gradually increase the depth and force of the movements as pain eases. Also use deep stroking actions with your fingertips along the length of the tendon (*see* fig 5.9, page 66).

EXERCISES

Exercise is used to stretch the tendon and load it. The ankle bending exercise on pages 46–47 may also be used to stretch the Achilles tendon. Place your foot flat on a chair seat and press your knee forwards. Hold the position for 30–60 seconds, without lifting your heel.

Achilles tendon stretch – standing

Purpose
To stretch the Achilles tendon over a prolonged period.

Preparation
Stand with your back up against a wall and have a block or thick book to hand.

Action
Place your toes on the book and allow your heels to lower down to the floor. Allow your knees to bend slightly (soften) to take some of the stretch from the calf muscles. Lean back against the wall

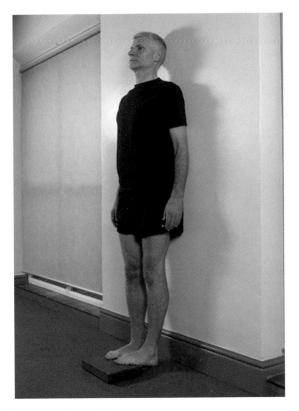

Figure 5.10 Achilles tendon stretch – standing

so you are not holding your calf muscles tensed. Hold the stretch for 2 minutes.

Tips
This action should not be intensely painful, but should give a pleasantly intense stretch. If you feel pain, use a lower block for 1 minute, rest and then use a slightly higher block for 1 minute.

Eccentric loading on the Achilles

Purpose
To encourage correct healing of the tendon tissue.

Preparation

Stand close to a step and have a small (2–3 kg) dumbbell to hand. Place your toes onto the step leaving your heels free.

Action

Rise up onto the toes of both feet. Transfer your bodyweight to your injured leg and then lower back to the starting position taking 10 seconds to do so. Repeat this action for 10 reps and then rest for 30 seconds. Perform 3–5 sets of this action twice daily. If you find the exercise does not work your Achilles hard, grasp the dumbbell in the hand opposite your injury (left Achilles affected, dumbbell in right hand) and lift using the weight.

Tips

Research has shown that the Achilles tendon tissue will change favourably with intense loading. To achieve this you may need to use a heavier weight. If you do not have dumbbells, use some food cans placed in a carrier bag or put them in a rucksack and wear this during your Achilles exercise.

As your Achilles pain eases you may return to sport gradually. In the case of running, use speed walking to begin and progress to scout pace (run-walk-run-walk). When you can do this without pain begin running short distances and build up over a period of days and weeks. Table 5.1 shows an example of a suitable progression. Timings are taken from the point of tolerable pain. The progression assumes that at no time does pain increase, and that running takes place only when pain no longer occurs. The hop and hold exercise described on page 64 may also be used to work the Achilles, training it for rapid actions.

Table 5.1	Exercise progression for Achilles tendinopathy
As pain eases, days 1–2	Slow walking, focussing on equal step length.
As pain eases, days 3–4	Reverse walking, sideways walking, cross leg (grapevine) walking.
Minimal pain, days 5–7	Power walk on flat, and then on inclined treadmill at 5% gradient, progressing to 10% gradient.
Minimal pain, days 8–14	Scout pace, walk-run-walk-run. Take 5 steps for each, progressing to 10 and then 15. Duration 2 minutes total, progressing to 5 minutes total.
No pain, days 15–21	Slow run on flat surface. Walk for 2 minutes followed by 5-minute run and 1-minute walk and reverse walk to finish. Progress flat run to 10 minutes then 15 minutes.
Week 4–5	Run on varying terrain. Walk for 2 minutes followed by 10 minute run on field or canal towpath. Progress run to 15–20 minutes.
Week 6–8	Alter running direction. Run straight to begin followed by slow reverse run, side step, zigzag and bend running. Walk to recover between each section. Duration 10–12 minutes total.
Week 9–12	Longer run introducing hills. Total of 20–30 minutes. Walk 2 minutes on flat to finish. Progress running time for distance runners and running speed for those in sports involving sprinting.
Months 4–6 building to normal training	Fartlek training. Walk, jog, run, short sprint, walk to recover. Flat and straight to begin, then introducing hills, zigzag, reverse running and rapid direction change at speed later.

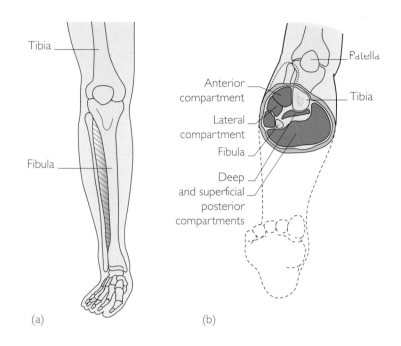

Figure 5.11 The shin: (a) shin muscles positioned along the shin bones (b) cross section showing muscle compartments

SHIN SPLINTS

Shin splints is a condition familiar to many distance runners, but it can actually occur in any sport involving running. The shin muscles are positioned along the shin bones (*tibia* and *fibula*), sandwiched between the flat bones on one side and the tight skin of the shin on the other (*see* fig 5.11). The various shin muscles are grouped together and each group is separated from the next by a tight membrane called *fascia*. This tight packaging is called a *compartment*, hence the official title of shin splints – *compartment syndrome*.

When you work any muscle it fills with blood (pumps up) and bulges. The same happens to the shin muscles, but, because they are constricted within tight compartments, there is less room for

them to bulge. The fascia which houses the muscles will give slightly over time and adapt to training, but not as fast as the muscle. If you suddenly increase the intensity of your training, or change it, the muscles pump up too quickly. As they try to bulge, their widthways expansion is restricted by the wall of the compartment they are in, and the pressure within the muscle increases like a sausage in a skin. The expanding pressure within the muscle causes the blood vessels which pass within to collapse, shutting off the blood flow to the muscle. Starved of oxygen, and no way of getting rid of its waste products, the muscles becomes very painful. In some cases (fortunately rare) the compartment is so tight and the muscle pressure builds up so quickly that the muscle will actually die. This requires immediate surgery to cut the restricting muscle compartment (an operation called a *fasciotomy*).

Your treatment should aim to reduce pain and pressure within the muscle and you should adapt your training programme to avoid the shin splints coming back. Initially, treatment is total rest from all sporting activity. During this time you can use massage to relieve pain and tension within the shin muscles, and taping to ease the condition in day-to-day activities. Before returning to your sport you must prepare the muscles, and this is where exercise therapy is used. We will focus mostly on pain at the front (anterior compartment) of the shin which affects the tibialis anterior muscle and toe extensors.

HEAT AND COLD

Use cold baths initially to ease any muscle swelling in the shins. This may be in a deep bowl or bath, and the water should have ice cubes in it. Soak the shins for 10–15 minutes twice daily. Ice massage used along the shin will help to reduce local swelling and improve circulation through the muscle.

As pain eases and tension within the shin resulting from local swelling reduces, hot packs used prior to massage and stretching. The packs should be comfortably warm, and you should monitor the shin two or three times throughout treatment to make sure you do not burn yourself. When the shins are painful they are often less sensitive to heat, so you may not feel a burn. Apply the hot pack for 15–20 minutes before going on to massage and/or stretching.

MASSAGE

Your partner should be sitting with their knees bent. General massage is performed using the fingers to stroke along the length of the muscle compartment. A cooling cream or rub containing peppermint essential oil is often very relieving.

Specific massage is now used to the precise site of pain. Deep pressure is required, and to save your fingers it is a good idea to use a massage tool. Where painful nodules (trigger points) are found, use sustained pressure to the area for 30–60 seconds until the pain subsides. Self-pressure may be applied using a golf ball or spiky ball. Stand close to a wall and place the spiky ball over the painful spot, sandwiched between the wall and your shin (*see* fig 5.12). Lean into the wall to press the ball into your shin and hold the position until pain eases. Using a spiky ball to massage along the painful shin stimulates the circulation.

TAPING

Taping (spiral deload taping) may be used to reduce the pull on the fascia within the shin and so relieve pain.

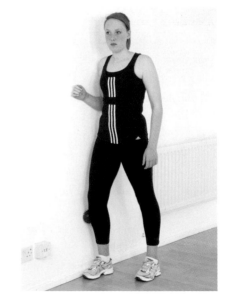

Figure 5.12 Specific massage using a spiky ball

- Begin by fixing the tape just above your outer ankle bone. Pull the tape lengthways to draw the shin up as you put the tape on.

- Where pain is on the front of the shin (anterior compartment syndrome), the tape goes across the front of the shin to the inside and then around the back of the calf to the outside of the shin again (*see* fig 5.13).

- Where pain is on the outside of the shin (lateral compartment syndrome), fix anchors above the outer ankle bone and below the outside of the knee.

- Place the end of a tape stirrup on the lower anchor and draw the tape upwards to fix it to the upper anchor. Two or three tape strips may be required.

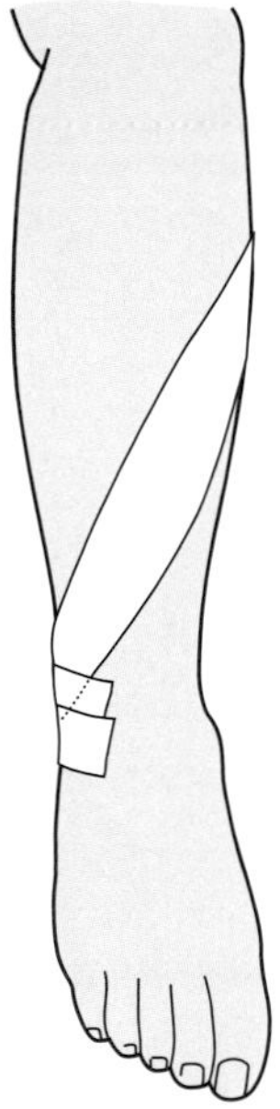

EXERCISES

Shin stretch – standing

Purpose

To lengthen the front (anterior) shin muscles and relieve pain.

Preparation

Begin standing, holding onto the back of a chair of piece of gym equipment. Place a folded towel on the floor.

Action

Point your ankle and toes, and press the front of your foot into the towel to straighten it. You should feel the stretch along the length of your shin muscles to the outside of the shin.

Figure 5.13 Taping for anterior compartment syndrome showing shin splint taping from the outside of the ankle around the front of the shin to the back of the calf

Tips

You may need to alter the angle of your foot by pressing it more onto the big toe side to feel the stretch specifically on your painful area.

Shin stretch – kneeling

Purpose

To lengthen the front (anterior) shin muscles over a prolonged period.

Preparation

You will need a yoga mat or thick folded towel and two or three yoga blocks (see fig 5.15, overleaf).

71

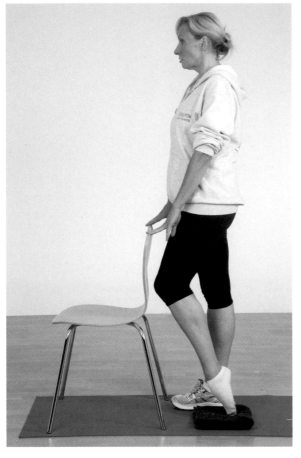

Figure 5.14 Shin stretch – standing

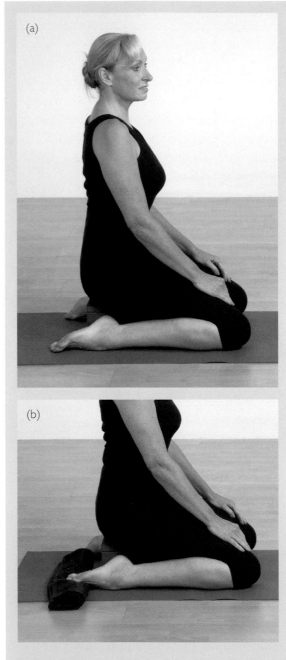

(a)

(b)

Figure 5.15 Shin stretch – kneeling

Action

With bare feet, kneel on the mat with your shins parallel and toes pointed behind you. Place the blocks between your feet. Gradually sit back towards your heels until your buttocks touch the blocks (*see* fig 5.15a). Sit in this position for 1–2 minutes until the tightness and pain in the shins eases. Remove one block and sit down further for another 1–2 minutes.

Tips

This stretch enables you to stretch your shins for a prolonged period and relax into the position. It also places a stretch on your knees and ankles. If these joints are very tight, use more blocks to reduce the stress on the knees, and place a folded towel beneath the front of your ankles to reduce the stress here (*see* fig 5.15b, page 72).

Toe raise walk

Purpose

To strengthen and build endurance in the front shin muscles.

Preparation

Begin standing with your feet hip width apart.

Action

Lift one foot to feel the shin muscles tighten, relax and then lift the other foot. Perform 10–20 reps of this alternating movement. Providing this is comfortable, lift your toes and walk forwards for 10–20 paces just on your heels. Rest for 2 minutes and then repeat.

Tips

Build up the time you can perform this exercise before pain comes on. Practise walking with the toes pointing forwards, then pointing outwards and then inwards.

Front shin strengthening using resistance

Purpose

To strengthen and pump up the front shin muscles to build muscle endurance.

Preparation

Begin sitting on a high bench or table. Place some cans or bottles in a carrier bag to act as resistance and hook it around your toes.

Action

Pull your foot up to tighten your shin muscles and then lower. Perform 30–50 reps, rest and then repeat (*see* fig 5.16, page 74).

Tips

Initially, the bag should touch the floor so you get a small rest between reps to allow some recovery. Progress to sitting higher so the bag does not touch the floor and tension is maintained in the muscle throughout the whole exercise period. This will build up the muscle tolerance to waste products and acids produced during exercise.

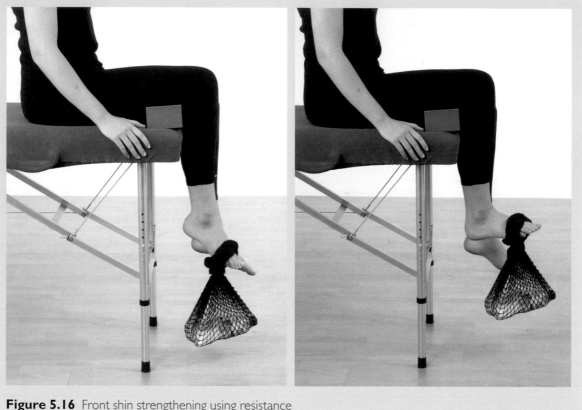

Figure 5.16 Front shin strengthening using resistance

When you return to sport do so progressively. Initially, run only twice or three times per week, and then every other day to allow your shin muscles to recover between training bouts. Try to vary your training rather than running for the same distance each week throughout the year. Use periodisation to split the year up, focusing for some months on distance work and some on fast pace running. Have a period when you lay off running and concentrate on weight training and stretching. This will allow your legs to recover from running but also work other aspects of your fitness.

Often one of the reasons that shin pain occurs is the alignment of your foot. It is a good investment to see a podiatrist or physiotherapist to get your foot alignment checked out, as orthotics (special shoe inserts) may be required.

Terms you should know:

Contrast bathing – immersing a body part in hot and cold water alternately, to increase blood flow.

Deload taping – tape positioned to take weight or stress of body tissues.

Fascia – a layer of fibrous tissue surrounding and connecting body structures including muscle, bone, organs and nerves. In several places the fascia may thicken and become specialised, for example the *fascia lata* on the outside (lateral aspect) of the thigh.

Overuse – an injury which develops slowly.

Periodisation – a method of splitting a training period up (weekly/monthly/yearly) to focus on different fitness components at a time and avoid overtraining.

Scout pace – a short period of running interspaced with a short period of walking. The run-walk-run-walk cycle is repeated continually.

Tendinopathy – general term for any disease of a tendon. It may include inflammation (tendonitis), degeneration, excess blood vessel growth (neovascularisation) and rupture.

Trauma – an injury which occurs suddenly.

6

// KNEE

The knee is essentially two joints. The knee joint is formed between the thigh bone (femur) and shin bone (tibia) and officially called the *tibiofemoral joint*. The kneecap joint lies between the thigh bone (femur) and kneecap (patella) and is called the *patellofemoral joint*. Going back into our prehistoric past, the knee joint was actually in two parts. Now, the two have united into a single joint, but we still have an inner and outer knuckle, each called a *condyle*. As with all major joints in the body, the knee contains fluid and is strengthened by ligaments (*see* fig 6.1). However, the knee is unique in that it has an extra set of

ligaments, deep inside, called the *cruciates*. The ligaments on the inside (medial) and outside (lateral) of the joint support the knee in side-to-side movements, while the cruciates support it in forward and backward movements (*see* fig 6.11, page 85).

MEDIAL LIGAMENT

The *medial ligament* is on the inside of the knee joint. It is a flat band about 8 cm long and consists of several parts. This structure enables a part of the ligament to remain tight to support the joint at all times, even when the knee is bent. Injury to the

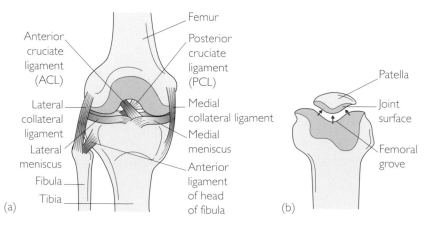

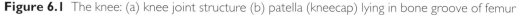

Figure 6.1 The knee: (a) knee joint structure (b) patella (kneecap) lying in bone groove of femur

medical ligament typically occurs when you twist your body but keep your foot planted on the ground. Sprain is common in sports such as football, and as you can imagine skiing is a common culprit as well. Pain occurs on the inside of the joint and you can straighten the knee, but find bending difficult. A therapist will normally test the joint by unlocking it slightly and bending the shin outwards slightly. This action tries to gap the inside of the joint, a movement normally protected by the medial ligament. If the ligament is injured, the action is painful. Mild injury (grade I or II) gives pain, but the joint is stable. A complete ligament rupture will allow the joint to open sideways and the joint is unstable. Often, however, with so much pain and protective muscle spasm, it is difficult to examine the joint by hand and a scan is needed.

> ### Keypoint
> Marked muscle spasm can cover up a ligament rupture, making a joint appear more stable than it actually is.

INITIAL TREATMENT

Where the ligament is very painful and you are unable to take weight on it, your knee must be protected in a brace and you should walk with crutches. As the knee heals, taping may be all that is required. To tape the knee, use non-elastic strip taping at the inside of the joint (*see* fig 6.2).

- Begin with the knee slightly bent (15 degrees) and apply two anchors, one above the knee and one below.

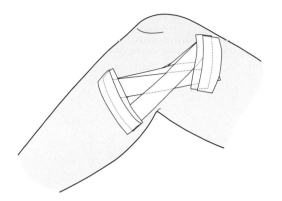

Figure 6.2 Medial ligament taping of the knee

- Tape stirrups are placed between the anchors, at an angle to each other to reinforce the joint as it bends.

- The taping will restrict your knee bending to about 20–30 degrees and give you some support as you walk.

If you are able to bend your knee more than 45 degrees without pain, a commercial knee support is better than taping.

Several elastic knee supports (*see* fig 6.3, overleaf) are available which are reinforced on the inside. These may be elasticated fabric or neoprene and normally Velcro-closed to give an adjustable compression. For further support, plastic or metal hinged stays are often placed on the inside of the brace. These are known as *functional supports*, because they protect the knee from actions which would stress the medial ligament, but allow other movements to occur.

An ice pack may be applied to the area to reduce inflammation. Avoid placing the ice directly on your skin as this may burn, especially over areas of prominent bone, where your skin is

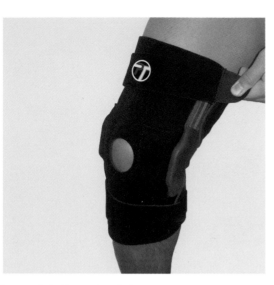

Figure 6.3 Example of a knee support

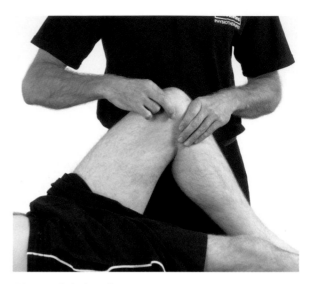

Figure 6.4 Specific massage to the medial ligament

stretched tightly and thinner. A commercial ice pack may be used, but when this is not to hand a frozen packet of peas from the home freezer makes a good alternative. To avoid the pack freezing to your skin, wrap it in a damp cloth or tea towel – the cloth protects your skin and the moisture allows the cold to get through. Leave the pack on for about 15 minutes and apply it 3 or 4 times each day for the two days immediately after injury, reducing to twice daily after that when the swelling will have normally stopped forming.

Keypoint

A frozen packet of peas makes a good alternative to a commercial ice pack for application to an injured area. To avoid the pack freezing to your skin, wrap it in a damp tea towel and apply for 15 minutes.

MASSAGE

Specific massage to the medial ligament is given with your partner lying with their injured knee bent. Circular frictions are used over the painful area, and deep transverse friction (DTF) applied to the ligament itself (*see* fig 6.4). Often the most painful portion is at the point where the two bones in the joint meet, an area called the *joint line*. This is on the inside of the knee at a level roughly the same as the lower part of your kneecap. Begin here performing slow circles of 1–2 cm to reduce pain and local swelling. For DTF, press more deeply so that your fingers and your partner's skin move as one. You should aim to sweep your fingers to and fro 15–20 times. This may be uncomfortable, but should not be very painful, and the discomfort should ease as you perform the massage. If the area becomes more painful, stop, because you may be irritating the tissues.

Self-massage is easily given by sitting with your knee bent and resting on a cushion to the side. You can massage deeply with your thumb

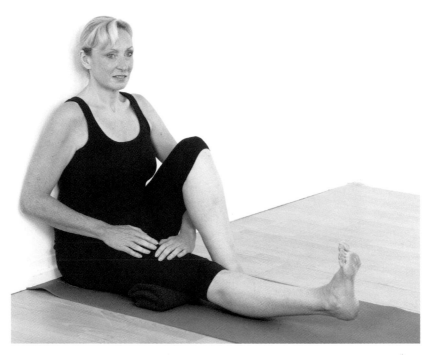

Figure 6.5 Quads bracing

for 30–60 seconds, bend and straighten your knee several times to recover, and then repeat the massage.

EXERCISES

After a knee injury the body responds by forcing you to rest. It does this by stopping your knee muscles from working, a process called *pain inhibition*. Although this is a primitive safeguard against continuing tissue damage, the process overacts. Exercise is vital initially to slow the process of muscle wasting and then to build up the muscles to stabilise your knee. Returning to sport on a knee with muscle wasting leaves the knee unprotected and open to further (and often more serious) injury.

Keypoint

Returning to sport with muscle wasting following an injury leaves your body unprotected and at risk to further injury.

Quads bracing

Purpose

To reduce muscle wasting following injury and encourage full knee bracing.

Preparation

Sit on the floor with your back supported against a wall. Place a folded towel beneath your knee.

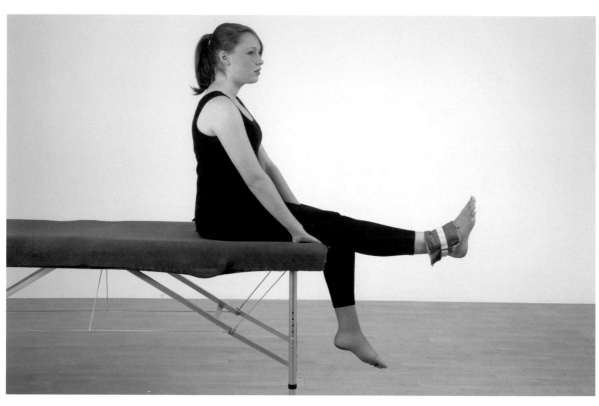

Figure 6.6 Leg extension

Action
Tighten your thigh muscles (quadriceps) to draw your kneecap up. Tighten once for 1–2 seconds and then relax slightly before tightening again harder. Relax, and repeat for a third time (*see* fig 6.5, page 79).

Tips
When muscles are not working properly it is often hard to switch them on. By tightening, and then relaxing partially before contracting again more intensely, you are often able to get a superior muscle contraction. Also try contracting your uninjured leg at the same time. The nervous impulses from this contraction with often spread (overflow) to your injured side.

Leg extension
Purpose
To re-strengthen the quads after injury.

Preparation
Begin sitting on a table or bedside with a weight bag (1–2 kg) hooked over your ankle.

Action
Draw your toes upwards and straighten your leg, locking your knee out fully (*see* fig 6.6). Perform

8–10 reps, rest for 1 minute and then repeat. Perform 3 sets of 8–10 reps each day for 1 week. Increase the weight (5–10 kg) for the second week and perform 3 sets of 8–10 reps every other day.

Tips

Pulling your toes towards you mimics the action of walking (heel strike), when your knee is normally locked out straight. This often helps you to contract the muscle fully after injury.

Mini squat

Purpose

To rehearse the natural action of knee straightening (functional knee locking).

Preparation

Begin standing facing a wall with your feet hip width apart. Optionally, you may perform this without a wall, standing feet hip-width apart.

Action

Bend your knees, keeping your trunk upright so that your hands slide down the wall by 20 cm. Pause for 1–2 seconds in the low position and then stand up again. Perform 8–10 reps. To progress the exercise make the balance harder by performing the mini squat with no support, away from the wall (*see* fig 6.7).

Tips

As you squat down aim to keep your kneecap over the centre of your foot. If your kneecap goes over the inside of your foot you are performing the squat with knock-knees. If your kneecap goes to the outside of your foot you are bow-legged. Both are examples of poor knee alignment.

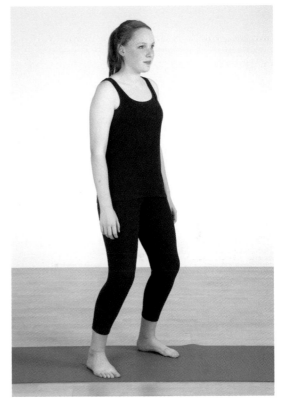

Figure 6.7 Mini squat

Knee stability

Purpose

To develop muscular stability and confidence in the knee.

Preparation

Begin standing on your injured leg by a wall (away from the wall for a harder exercise). Bend (soften) your knee slightly.

Action

Initially, try to stand on one leg without holding the wall and without wobbling for 20–30 seconds. Once you have achieved this try the same action

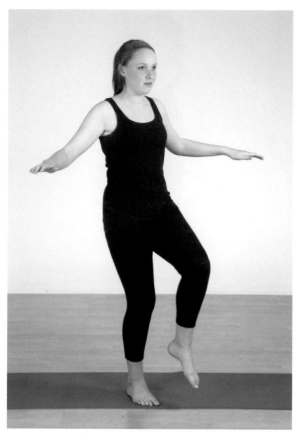

Figure 6.8 Knee stability

KNEECAP PAIN

Pain around the kneecap is common in teenagers and later in life with active seniors. The condition is officially called *patellofemoral pain syndrome* (PFPS) and results from a change in the way the kneecap moves. The kneecap is triangular in cross section and sits in a shallow groove on the lower portion of the thighbone (femur) (*see* fig 6.11, page 85). The cap essentially floats, having no bony connection. It is held in place by the strong thigh muscles (quadriceps) above and a strong tendon below. At each side there is thick tissue called the *retinaculum*, which stops the kneecap from moving sideways, towards or away from the body.

As you bend and straighten your knee, your kneecap moves up and down (tracks) and should stay in the centre of the bone groove of the thighbone. To do this, there must be equal forces acting on the inside and outside edges of the kneecap. These forces come from three sources: first, the pull of your thigh muscles; second, the tightness of the retinaculum attaching to the kneecap; and, third, the position of your foot and the twisting effect that this can cause on the leg bone. One or all of these three factors must be addressed when you get pain.

> **Keypoint**
>
> For the kneecap to be positioned correctly within the bone groove of the thighbone, the forces acting on the cap must be balanced. Unbalanced forces force the kneecap to deviate from its optimal movement path (maltracking).

with your eyes closed for the same time. Open your eyes and turn (rotate) your body from side to side for 10 reps while maintaining your balance and knee alignment – your kneecap should be positioned over the centre of your foot (*see* fig 6.8).

Tips

The function of the medial ligament is to support the knee in twisting and side-to-side actions. With this exercise you are building up your muscles to help with this function and so take some strain off the ligament.

If the kneecap fails to stay in the centre of its groove as you move, it can scrape the groove at one side causing swelling and pain. In addition, by moving to one side, the tissues on one side of the knee will be overstretched giving pain. This all occurs slowly, so you often notice pain after sitting for a long time and the knee seems to take time to get going. Also, the more stress that is put on the knee, the more pain you will get. People often complain of pain going down steps or coming downhill rather than going up. This is because the forces acting on the knee are greater.

HOT AND COLD PACKS

When you get pain over the kneecap, rest is needed initially to allow the condition to settle. This can be helped by gentle warmth over the knee from a microwaveable hot pack. The increase in blood flow and the gentle numbing effect of the warmth will often give enough pain relief to allow you to perform your day-to-day activities. If there is swelling around the kneecap, use an ice pack instead. This will settle the swelling, and again has a numbing effect. Some people do not like cold over their kneecap, however, and often feel that it stiffens the knee and makes the condition worse. There is some scientific evidence for this. Laboratory experiments using heat photographing cameras (thermal imaging) have shown that this condition often has a reduced blood flow to the kneecap, and it is probably this that you feel when you do not like the thought of anything cold on your knee.

TAPING

Taping can be used to gently draw the kneecap to one side and correct its faulty position (patella alignment).

- Because the skin over the kneecap is delicate you should use two types of taping. The first is a mesh which sticks to your skin quite gently (*see* fig 6.9a, page 84).

- On top of this you put a strong adhesive tape and pull it inwards (*see* fig 6.9b, page 84). The inward pull helps reposition the kneecap and take some of the excessive stretch from the tissues which can be the cause of your pain.

- Don't worry that the tape creases when you do this. Normally creasing of the tape can lead to skin irritation, but in this taping procedure we have protected the skin with mesh specifically to prevent this.

- The taping should reduce the pain around the kneecap as you move your knee. If your pain increases, take the taping off, because you need a physiotherapist to assess your condition closely and teach you a taping technique individually designed for your knee.

EXERCISES

Knee alignment
Purpose
To correct faulty knee alignment during bending activities.

Preparation
Wearing shorts, stand on a hard floor in bare feet. Your feet should be hip width apart.

Action
Take your weight onto the outside of your feet increasing the height of your foot arches, and

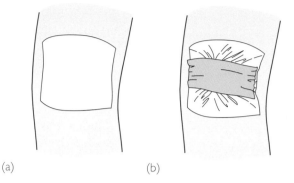

(a)   (b)

Figure 6.9 Patella taping: (a) non-elastic taping is placed over fibrous net for skin protection (b) shows the drag on skin

then onto the inside of your feet to reduce the arch height. As you do so, notice your kneecaps moving inwards and outwards. Stop in the position where your kneecaps point forwards rather than out or in.

Tips
If you find your foot naturally rests flat, you should wear training shoes to support your arches and use an orthotic in your day-to-day footwear.

Self-monitored knee alignment
Purpose
To strengthen the front thigh muscles (quads) while maintaining optimal knee alignment.

Preparation
Begin standing barefooted wearing shorts. Using a felt pen, draw a vertical line through the centre of your kneecap, and a line on your foot extending back from your third toe.

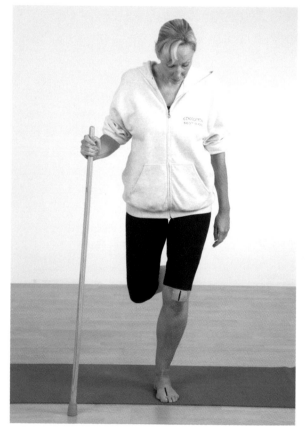

Figure 6.10 Self-monitored knee alignment

Action

Look down at your kneecap and position your knee so the line on your kneecap is directly over the line on your foot (*see* fig 6.10, page 84). Bend and straighten your knee to 30 degrees, keeping this alignment.

Tips

It sometimes helps to close one eye when you look down at the two lines.

Step down

Purpose

To strengthen the front thigh muscles (quads) using controlled muscle lengthening (eccentric action).

Preparation

Stand on your injured leg on a low step or block.

Action

Keep your pelvis level (do not allow it to sag down on one side) and bend your knee slowly, keeping your knee over the centre of your foot. Put both feet back on the step and stand up using both legs. Repeat the action for 10 reps, lowering with one leg and lifting back up with both.

Tips

To progress this exercise slow down the lowering portion taking 10–15 seconds.

CRUCIATES

The *cruciates* are extra ligaments inside your knee. There are two: the *anterior cruciate ligament* (ACL), which is more commonly injured, and the *posterior cruciate ligament* (PCL) (*see* fig 6.11). The cruciates help to stop your thigh bone from sliding forwards and backwards on top of your shin bone. When the ACL is torn, the medical test is to try to move one bone on the other either with the hands or with a special machine called an *arthrometer*, which detects very small movements. ACL injury normally occurs during an accident involving considerable force, such as

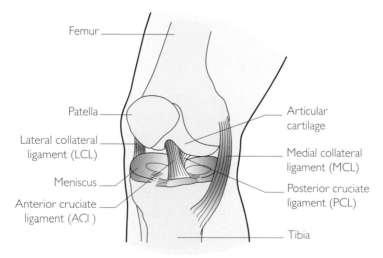

Figure 6.11 The major ligaments of the knee

Femur
Patella
Lateral collateral ligament (LCL)
Meniscus
Anterior cruciate ligament (ACL)
Articular cartilage
Medial collateral ligament (MCL)
Posterior cruciate ligament (PCL)
Tibia

skiing, falling from a horse, or falling and twisting the knee while running. Often, other structures in the knee may be injured as well. In the worst case scenario the ACL is injured together with the inner knee cartilage (meniscus) and inner knee ligament (MCL). This very serious combination of injuries is called an *unhappy triad* and can end a player's career.

Minor cruciate tears can be treated using exercise therapy, but more major injury requires surgery followed by intensive exercise therapy later. Exercise can be effective because the cruciates are only one structure which stops the thigh and shin bones sliding on top of each other. Your muscles also support the knee, and nowadays less surgery is done for minor ACL tears because exercise for this type of injury can be more effective.

Where the ACL is surgically repaired, either a false ligament is put in, or one of your other tendons (normally the hamstrings or a piece of patellar tendon) is diverted into the knee to do the job of the ACL. After such surgery it can take 6–12 months for the knee to fully recover, and recovery is dependent on correct exercise.

Often after knee injury we are concerned with muscle strength. This is because the knee muscles can waste when the knee is injured and swollen. Although strength is important after ACL injury as well, we are more concerned with the knee being stable and not giving way. This is a function of muscle speed because your knee muscles have to contract quickly enough to support your knee before it gives out. You may have very strong knee muscles, but if they don't contract quickly, your knee may still be unstable. To train knee muscle speed we use balance exercises rather than just ones for strength.

> **Keypoint**
> Joint stability depends not just on muscle strength, but on muscle contraction speed as well.

EXERCISES

Balance – standing
Purpose
To redevelop muscular stability of the knee.

Preparation
Begin standing holding onto the top of a chair.

Action
Stand on your injured leg, unlock your knee by bending it 5–10 degrees and maintain this balance. Let go of the chair back, first with one hand and then the other. Hold the single leg standing position for 20–30 seconds, rest and then repeat.

Tips
Keep your pelvis correctly aligned – do not dip your hip on your injured side.

Knee stability on a balance disc
Purpose
To progress muscular stability of the knee.

Preparation
Begin standing on a balance disc holding the top of a chair.

Action
Gradually bend and straighten your knee by 10–15 degrees, trying to keep the edge of the balance disc

off the floor. Perform 10 reps, rest and then repeat, holding the chair with just one hand.

Tips
Keep looking forwards – do not look at your feet.

Slide training
Purpose
To train the knee to withstand shearing (horizontal) forces.

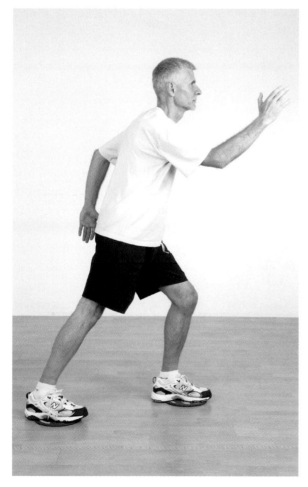

Figure 6.12 Slide training

Preparation
Begin standing on a polished wooden floor. You may also use a commercially available slide trainer or slide disc (*see* fig 6.12).

Action
Keep your knee unlocked (soft). Slowly slide your foot forwards and backwards for 5 reps, and then side to side for 5 reps. Rest and repeat, moving your leg slightly faster (*see* fig 6.12).

Tips
Vary the length of your sliding stride, moving by 10–20 cm for some reps and 30–40 cm for others.

Hop and hold
Purpose
To build knee stability and control.

Preparation
Stand in the gym in an open space away from equipment.

Action
Hop forwards on your injured leg by 10–20 cm. Hold the position for 1–2 seconds and then hop again. Repeat for 10 reps. Rest and then practise hoping sideways, backwards and in a zigzag using the same rhythm.

Tips
The hold is performed in the landing position to gain control over single leg balance. To progress the exercise, reduce the holding period and increase the hoping distance.

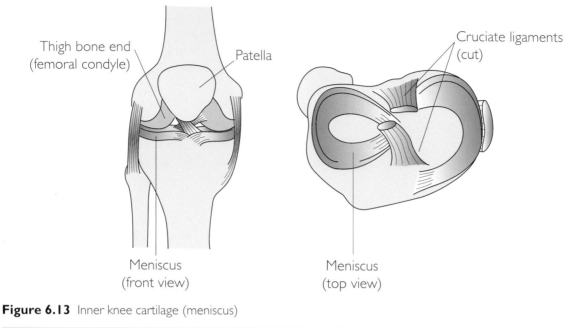

Thigh bone end
(femoral condyle)

Patella

Cruciate ligaments
(cut)

Meniscus
(front view)

Meniscus
(top view)

Figure 6.13 Inner knee cartilage (meniscus)

KNEE CARTILAGE

In most of your joints, the ends of the bones are covered by a layer of cartilage. In the knee, however, there are two additional cartilage structures each called a *meniscus*. These are crescent-shaped structures which are wider on the outside and thinner towards the centre (*see* fig 6.13). The outer edge of the meniscus is attached to the shin bone via the thin coronary ligament. There is a meniscus on the outside of the knee (lateral meniscus) and one on the inside (medial meniscus) (*see* fig 6.1a, page 76). Their function is to distribute weight more evenly across the ends of the bones. Because the ends are rounded, the area of contact between the bones is quite small. By having the menisci, the contact area is made larger.

The most common injury to the knee menisci is a tear to the medial meniscus (*see* fig 6.13). This usually occurs when your foot is planted firmly on the ground and you twist your body: the combination of stationary shin bone and moving thigh bone while supporting your whole bodyweight can tear the meniscus. The tear can be of several types. The meniscus can split in its centre, or an end can tear off the underlying bone. Sometimes it is just the edge of the meniscus which is damaged.

If just the very edge of the meniscus and its coronary ligament attachment is injured, it may heal through rest. This is because the outer edge of the structure has a blood supply. The inner part of the meniscus does not have a blood supply, so when it is injured it must be surgically repaired or removed.

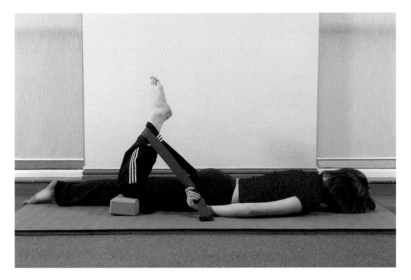

Figure 6.14 Assisted knee bending

One of the key signs of injury to the meniscus is that the loose part of damaged tissue can hang freely between the knee bones, causing the knee to give way. When this happens the knee bones aren't able to come together fully, and the knee does not lock out straight. Because the knee cannot lock out properly, just when you rely on your knee to support you it suddenly buckles and you stumble or fall. Following injury the knee swells quickly and is very painful. As the pain and swelling subside, the knee does not recover and gives way when you least expect it. This is often when your attention is elsewhere, for example when stepping down from a step or turning suddenly to talk to someone.

Your physiotherapist will examine your knee and refer you to an orthopaedic surgeon. Treatment is usually through a keyhole operation and you will be left with several very small scars. Following surgery your rehabilitation begins. Start with an exercise such as quads bracing (page 79) and then progress to the assisted knee bending exercise detailed below.

> **Keypoint**
> If the knee cannot straighten fully (lock out) it may give way when you take weight through it.

EXERCISES

Assisted knee bending
Purpose
To reduce stiffness in your knee following swelling and/or surgery.

Preparation
Have a yoga belt (or towel) to hand and lie on your front on the floor. Bend your injured knee and

loop the band around your ankle and hold the band with both hands.

Action

Bend your knee as far as you can and then gently pull on the band to help the knee bend further. Hold the point of maximum bend (flexion) for 10–20 seconds and then release. Perform 5 reps and then walk around for 2–3 minutes to relax your knee before repeating.

Tips

As you are stretching a joint which is tight, expect this exercise to be slightly painful. On a scale of 1 (no pain) to 10 (maximum pain), you should not score more than 5–6, and pain should reduce as you are able to bend your knee further. If pain is more intense (7–10) or increases when you repeat the action, stop.

Lunge
Purpose
To develop leg strength and control.

Preparation
Begin standing with your feet shoulder width apart. Step forwards with your injured leg by about 1 m.

Action
Keep your trunk straight (do not lean forwards). Bend your leading (front) leg to 90 degrees, bringing the knee of your trailing (back) leg down towards the ground (*see* fig 6.15). Pause in the lower position and then press back up to standing. Perform 5 reps and then rest.

Tips
If you are unable to lower your body very far, or find that you wobble and lose your balance, place

one hand on a chair or table to stabilise yourself. Alternatively, hold a pole in one hand and use the pole for balance.

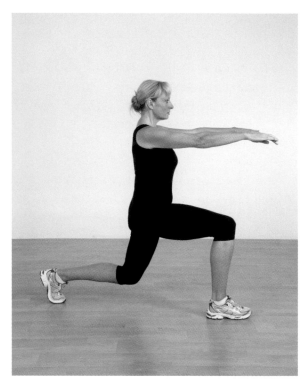

Figure 6.15 Lunge

QUADRICEPS TEAR

The *quadriceps* or 'quads' are a group of four muscles on the front of the thigh. Three of the muscles (together called the *vasti*) just work over the knee to straighten and lock it out straight. A fourth muscle – *rectus femoris* – is known as the *kicking muscle* and has this same action on the knee, but also works over the hip to bend it. Because the rectus muscle works over both the knee and hip joints, its action is more complex, and it is more commonly injured with rapid kicking and sprinting actions. In addition to tearing, the quads are also commonly bruised, being at the front of the thigh and therefore a contact point in many sports. Local quads bruising (contusion) can cause muscle spasm, giving rise to a 'deadleg' or 'charley horse' injury, where the muscle is so painful that the knee cannot be moved.

The treatment of a quads tear is the same as that for any other muscle, with one exception. With the quads there is a danger of the muscle healing with small calcium (bone) deposits within it – a medical condition called *myositis* (myositis ossificans). This can occur following a bad tear or extensive bruising when a player returns to sports too soon trying to 'play through the pain'. The first 24 hours after injury are the most dangerous period. To avoid myositis developing, it is important not to perform any sport in this period until the knee is able to bend to a right angle (90 degrees knee flexion), proving that the muscle is regaining its flexibility.

> ### Keypoint
> Following severe quads bruising, do not perform moderate or intense exercise until you can bend your knee to 90 degrees.

INITIAL TREATMENT

Bruising and swelling is limited by cold and compression. This can most easily be combined using a cold pack secured to the thigh using an elasticated bandage. Several commercially available cold bandages are also available which are impregnated with the same gel as the cold packs. In most cases it is more comfortable to rest with the knee straight, but when there is little bruising the thigh may be rested with the knee

bent to avoid the muscle going into spasm. Sit with the leg out straight and then bend the knee only to the position of maximum pain-free stretch, securing the pack to the leg by wrapping the bandage around both the thigh and shin.

TAPING

Taping for a quads tear may be used to limit excessive stretch and offer some support.

* Mesh underwrap is applied to the thigh initially.

* Elastic adhesive tape is then placed stretched along the length of the muscle (longitudinal taping) (*see* fig 6.16a, page 92).

* As the tape recoils it will feel tight on the thigh and remind you not to overstretch.

* Where compression rather than support is required, the elastic tape may be placed around the circumference of the leg to surround the thigh (transverse taping) (*see* fig 6.16b, page 92). This will restrict the formation of the bruising.

EXERCISES

Quads contraction through range
Purpose
To work the quads muscles throughout their whole range of motion.

Preparation
Attach a resistance band around the ankle of your injured leg. Lie on your back on a bench or firm bed (*see* fig 6.17a, page 92). Shuffle to the side so your injured leg hangs over the bench side,

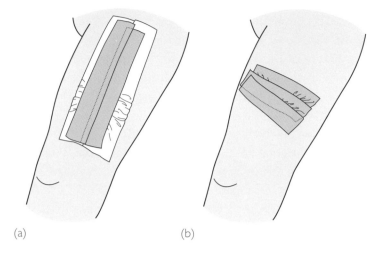

(a)   (b)

Figure 6.16 Quads taping: (a) longitudinal to prevent muscle overstretch (b) transverse

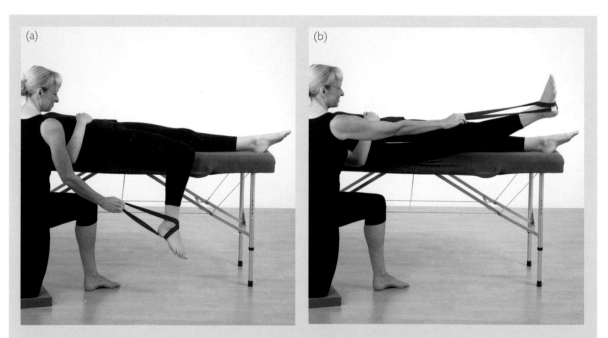

Figure 6.17 Quads contraction through range: (a) start position (b) knee extension

knee bent. Either have your training partner hold the free end of the band or tie it to the bench leg at the head end.

Action
Straighten your knee and at the same time lift your leg upwards off the couch by 15–20 cm (combined hip flexion and knee extension) (*see* fig 6.17b, page 92).

Tips
This exercise works both the upper and lower portions of the rectus femoris muscle as well as the other quads (vasti). Initially, the movement should be performed slowly. Later the movement can be performed more quickly, becoming a kicking action.

Quads stretch
Purpose
To stretch the whole of the quads at both the knee and the hip.

Preparation
Begin standing holding onto a chair or piece of gym equipment for balance.

Action
Bend the knee of your injured leg and catch hold of your ankle. Pull your heel towards your buttock and draw your knee further back than your hip (*see* fig 6.18).

Tips
Tighten your abdominals to prevent your pelvis tilting and your low back hollowing.

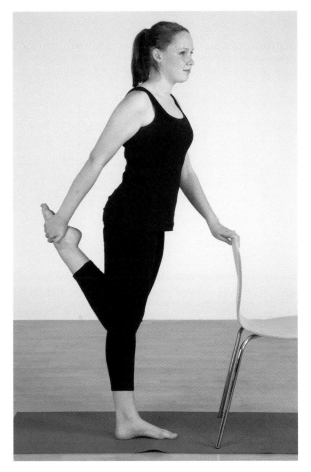

Figure 6.18 Quads stretch

Terms you should know:

ACL – anterior cruciate ligament of knee.

Arthrometer – medical device for measuring and recording joint movement.

Contraction speed – how fast a muscle can develop (maximal) force.

Deadleg – severe thigh muscle (quads) bruising combined with muscle spasm.

Maltracking – faulty movement of the kneecap.

Medial ligament – inner ligament of the knee consisting of several bands.

Myositis – medical condition where calcium is deposited within a muscle after injury.

Overflow – nervous impulses travelling to an injured muscle because the good muscle on the other side of the body is worked hard.

PCL – posterior cruciate ligament of the knee.

Retinaculum – strong fibrous band attaching between structures.

Thermal imaging – taking a photograph of heat rather than light.

Tracking – direction of movement of the kneecap within the groove of the thighbone.

HIP AND PELVIS

7

The hip is a ball and socket joint, with the ball (femoral head) at the end of the thighbone and the socket (acetabulum) within the pelvis. The hip and pelvis are therefore intimately linked, with pain in one usually involving the other.

HIP JOINT IMPINGEMENT

As the hip moves, the ball of the joint must remain in the centre of the socket. This is achieved through the balance of strength and flexibility of the powerful muscles surrounding the joint. Where muscle imbalance exists, the joint may be pulled out of alignment. The most common movement fault is for the joint to move forwards slightly (anterior impingement), giving pain in the groin and upper hip as the knee is brought towards the chest or lifted from the floor from a sitting position. This action is brought about through the action of the hip flexor muscles, which, as well as lifting the knee, pull the ball of the socket forwards. Normally, this would be balanced by deeper hip muscles which draw the ball backwards (gluteus medius and quadratus femoris), but, because we spend a lot of time sitting, the hip flexor muscles tend to be strong and short. Several exercises can be used to restore balance to the hip and correct this condition. Where pain remains after performing the exercises, you need to see a physiotherapist, who can monitor the position of your hip bones as you move.

> ### Keypoint
> Hip impingement can occur if the ball of the hip joint moves out of precise alignment with the hip socket. Muscle imbalance is a significant factor in this process.

EXERCISES

Rockback – kneeling
Purpose
To combine hip bending (flexion) with backwards glide of the hip joint ball (posterior femoral glide).

Preparation
Begin kneeling on a mat on all fours, with your knees shoulder width apart (*see* fig 7.1a, page 96).

Action
Press with your hands to rock your trunk backwards towards your heels (*see* fig 7.1b, page

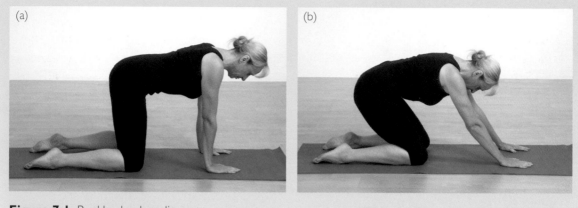

Figure 7.1 Rockback – kneeling

96). Go only as far as you can without getting hip pain. Perform 5 reps, rest 30 seconds and then repeat.

Tips
The aim of this exercise is to move comfortably without experiencing hip pain, rather than to stretch the knees. Stop the exercise when your buttocks are still off your heels.

Clamshell
Purpose
To strengthen and shorten the outer hip muscles (gluteus medius).

Preparation
Begin lying on your side with your knees bent and feet together. For comfort you may place a folded towel between your feet.

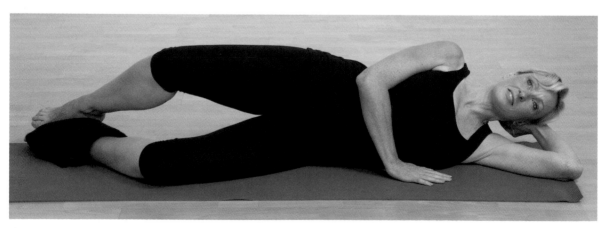

Figure 7.2 Clamshell

Action

Keeping your pelvis still, raise the knee of your top leg as far as possible (*see* fig 7.2, page 96). Pause in the upper position for 2–5 seconds and then lower. Perform 5 reps, rest and then repeat.

Tips

There is often a tendency to roll the pelvis back and twist the spine. If you find it difficult to keep you trunk fixed, perform the exercise with your buttocks against a wall.

Knee lift – sitting

Purpose

To re-educate the knee lifting action.

Preparation

Begin sitting on the edge of a firm chair with your knees and hips at 90 degrees, feet shoulder width apart. Place the fingers of one hand over the front of your hip joint within your groin.

Action

Press downwards with your fingers and lift your knee by 5–10 cm so that your foot clears the floor. Do not stop in the top position, but repeat 5 reps moving rhythmically.

Tips

Where you experience pain or discomfort through hip impingement, this action should reduce the pain.

SACROILIAC JOINT

The *sacroiliac joint* (SIJ) is the junction between the spine and the pelvis. The end of the spine is made up of a triangular-shaped bone, the *sacrum* (*see* fig 7.3, page 98). This has two flat joints, each of which joins onto one side of the pelvis, forming the SIJ. The weight of the body is taken through the spine and divided between the two legs at the SIJ. Normally, the SIJ moves very little, giving slightly during trunk and leg movements to avoid the area being brittle. However, the SIJ is held together by strong ligaments and these become soft during pregnancy as a result of female hormones. These hormones remain in the body for some months after childbirth, and are also released during menstruation each month, meaning that the SIJ moves more and is susceptible to injury at this time. In both sexes the SIJ can suffer from a sudden impact in jumping or slipping, causing the joint and surrounding tissues to inflame.

Keypoint

Female hormones released during pregnancy and menstruation enable the sacroiliac joint (SIJ) to move more.

The SIJ has very few muscles directly controlling it, but tendon material (fascia) from several muscles supports it. The gluteal, trunk and latissimus muscles and the hamstrings all provide stability to the SIJ. A number of self-treatments may be used, including SIJ belts, traction, self-mobilisation and stability work. General back stability work is covered in chapter 8.

SIJ BELT

The pelvis forms a ring, with the pubic joint at the front and the SIJs at the back. The sacrum bone forms a keystone in the ring. When the SIJ is painful, pain spreads into the buttock and often

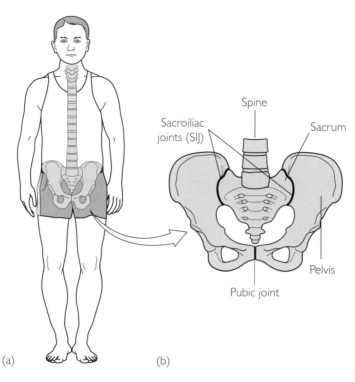

Figure 7.3 Hip and pelvis: (a) spine (b) pelvis and sacroiliac joints

down the leg. The pain typically gets worse when you stand for prolonged periods, especially when you favour one leg or stand on one leg alone. This illustrates that the SIJ may lack stability and using an SIJ belt may help. This belt is a strong webbing and elastic structure which wraps around the pelvis and is Velcro-closed at the front. It should be positioned around the sharp lip of the pelvis (anterior superior iliac spine) and not over the hip bone (greater trochanter). Pressure from the belt brings the ring of the pelvis together giving support.

EXERCISES

Door frame self-traction
Purpose
To reduce pain from SIJ and low back conditions.

Preparation
Begin standing in front of a door frame. Stand on a box or low chair if you are unable to reach the top rail (head) of the frame.

Action
Grip the rail with your fingertips and slowly bend your knees to stretch (traction) your spine. Hold the position for 30–60 seconds and then slowly release.

Tips

You are not aiming to take your full bodyweight, but to unload the spine by 2–5 lbs only. It is important to begin and end the movement slowly to avoid jolting the pelvis or spine.

Pelvic rock – standing

Purpose

To free off (mobilise) the pelvic joints and reduce pain.

Preparation

Begin standing with your back to a wall.

Action

Stand on one leg on your injured side. Lift your knee using your hands and gently pull it up to your chest and squeeze it in tightly to your ribs. Release until your knee is 5–10 cm from your chest and then reapply the squeezing action. Perform 5–10 reps as pain allows. Hold the knee as you lower it back to the floor.

Tips

You must support your leg weight throughout the whole exercise to avoid stress on the pelvis. The squeezing action places a small stress on the pelvic joints which, when repeated rhythmically, frees off the joints. As long as pain reduces you may continue, but if pain increases see a physiotherapist for a pelvic assessment.

Hip hinge with a pole

Purpose

To stabilise the pelvis and low back during bending.

Preparation

Begin standing with your feet hip width apart. Place a pole (broom handle) along the length of your spine, holding the top with one hand over your head and the bottom with the other hand beneath your tailbone.

Action

Bend your knees slightly (unlock them) and tip your body forwards, keeping your spine straight. Angle forwards to 45 degrees and then lift back up again (*see* fig 7.4b, overleaf). Perform 5–10 reps and then rest.

Tips

Your spine should stay aligned throughout the movement. If you hollow your back too much the lower part will come away from the stick markedly (*see* fig 7.4a, overleaf), and if you round it your shoulders will come off the stick (*see* fig 7.4b, overleaf). The alignment of your spine when you were standing at the beginning should be maintained throughout the exercise.

GROIN PAIN

There are several causes of pain in the groin (*see* fig 7.5, overleaf). The most common is strain to the adductor muscles (*adductor strain*), which function to close your legs. These muscles attach onto the pubic bones, and in some cases the bones themselves can be affected by a condition called *osteitis pubis*. An X-ray is needed if this condition is suspected by a physiotherapist. The X-ray normally shows mild bone density change to the region, with widening of the pubic joint (*pubic symphysis*).

Pain slightly higher up in the groin itself can come from a *sporting hernia*. This is overstretching and inflammation of the deep abdominal muscles where they attach to the top of the pelvis through

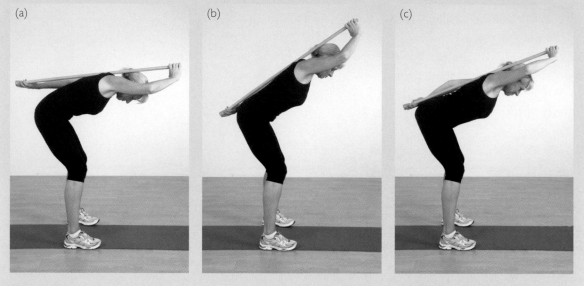

Figure 7.4 Hip hinge with a pole: (a) incorrect – spine bending (b) start position (c) forward angle

a specialised ligament (*inguinal ligament*). The sporting hernia requires rest initially, followed by training modification to address muscle imbalance. Typically, the condition is seen where the hip muscles are tight and you have performed too much abdominal work in training – such as sit-ups, trunk curls and crunches – without balancing this out with core stability (*see* chapter 8, page 129). By stretching the tight hips, reducing repeated abdominal work and focusing on core work the condition often resolves. In severe cases where physiotherapy has failed (3–6 months of rehab), the condition may require surgical repair.

Adductor strain affects the long adductor muscles, which attach into the pubic bones (*see* fig 7.5). There is normally pain in stretching and when adducting (closing) the leg against a resistance. Sit with your knees bent and place a ball between your knees. Squeeze the ball to see if this brings on your

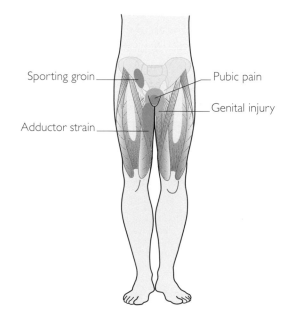

Figure 7.5 Location of groin pain

groin pain. Use your fingers to find the painful spot, and you can normally find a tight cord at the top of the groin going towards your pubic bone. This is the cord-like tendon of the adductor muscles. Initially, you should rest from any sport or daily activity which is painful. Self-massage and exercise can help to free the area off.

MASSAGE

To perform self-massage of the adductors, begin sitting on the floor with your legs out straight. Cross you injured leg over your uninjured one just above your knee. Allow your bent knee to drop down to the floor and place a cushion beneath your knee to take the weight of your leg. Apply some oil or massage cream to your skin and then massage the inside of your thigh, starting from the knee working up towards the groin bone. Use light and then deeper strokes to relax the muscle. Next, work into the muscles more deeply using circular actions with your fingertips. Again, work along the length of the adductor muscles from knee to groin bone. Finally, use deep transverse frictions (DTF) to the adductor tendons (*see* chapter 2, page 18). Press into your skin at the painful level of the tendon and work your fingers to and fro across the tendon, moving your fingers and thigh skin at the same time. Remember, when using DTF your fingers do not move *across* the skin, but *with* the skin (*see* fig 7.6).

EXERCISES

Figure-four knee lift
Purpose
To begin groin strengthening.

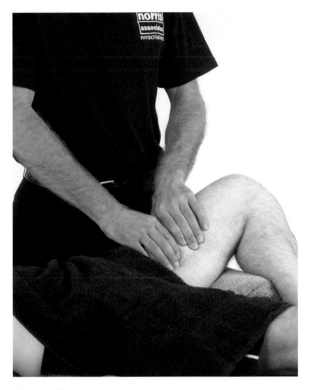

Figure 7.6 Adductor massage

Preparation
Sit on the floor with your legs out straight. Bend your injured leg over your uninjured one, crossing them above your knee to form a figure four.

Action
Allow your knee to lower towards the floor so that your thigh is horizontal. Pause in the lower position and then lift your knee until your thigh is vertical. Perform 10 reps and then repeat.

Tips
To increase the intensity of this exercise, place a 1–2 kg weight bag around your knee.

Groin stretch

Purpose
To stretch the adductor muscles.

Preparation
Begin sitting on the floor in bare feet. Bend your knees and place the soles of your feet together. You may wish to sit against a wall for support.

Action
Hold your feet using your cupped hands from beneath. Press your knee downwards and at the same time place overpressure onto your legs with your elbows. Exhale as you put the stretch on (do not hold your breath) and perform 5 reps, holding each stretch for 10 seconds.

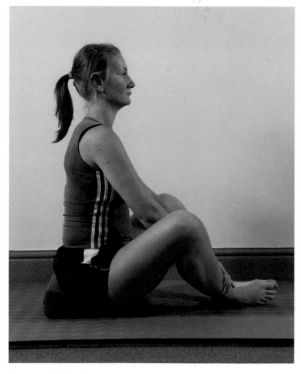

Figure 7.7 Groin stretch

Tips
Try to lengthen your spine and keep good alignment. If your back rounds and your pelvis rolls back (posterior pelvic tilt), the stretch is reduced at the groin. To prevent the pelvis rolling back, place a folded towel beneath your sitting bones (ischial tuberosities).

Straight leg groin stretch against a wall

Purpose
To stretch the long adductor muscle (adductor longus).

Preparation
Begin lying on the floor with your knees bent and buttocks against a wall.

Action
Straighten your legs so they are vertical and rest them against the wall (*see* fig 7.8a, page 103). Gradually lower them out to the sides (hip abduction) (*see* fig 7.8b, page 103). Hold in the lower position for 15–20 seconds and then bring your legs back to the vertical. Perform 3–5 reps.

Tips
This action combines hip adductor muscle contraction (pulling the feet together) with muscle stretch (moving the feet apart) and as such is a very effective type of stretching called *PNF* (proprioceptive neuromuscular facilitation). For more details of this type of stretching see *The Complete Guide to Stretching* (3rd edition) by Christopher Norris published by A&C Black (2007).

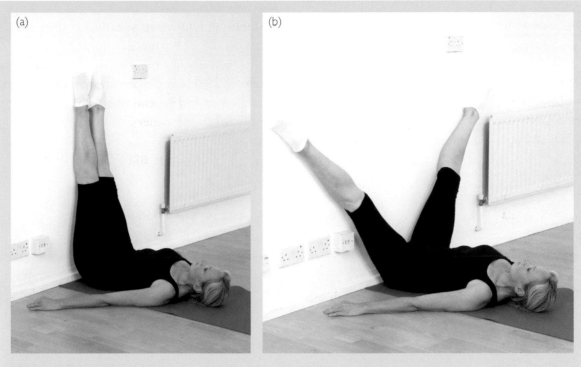

Figure 7.8 Straight leg groin stretch (a) start position (b) mid position

ITB SYNDROME

The *illiotibial band* (ITB) is a very strong, flat tendon-like tissue stretching down the side of your leg from the outside of your hip to the outside of your knee (*see* fig 7.9, page 104). It attaches to the crest of the pelvis and from here several gluteal muscles feed into it. The ITB stretches down the side of the leg appearing as a shallow groove on individuals with good muscular definition. At the knee it attaches to the outside of the shin bone (tibia), with some of its deep fibres stretching to the outside of the

kneecap. As the ITB descends from the pelvis to the side of the knee it passes over two prominent pieces of bone, one on the outside of the hip (greater trochanter) and the other on the outside of the knee (lateral epicondyle of the femur). If tight, the ITB can flick over these points like a guitar string, causing friction and pain. This painful condition is called *ITB friction syndrome* when it occurs at the hip and *runner's knee* when it occurs at the knee.

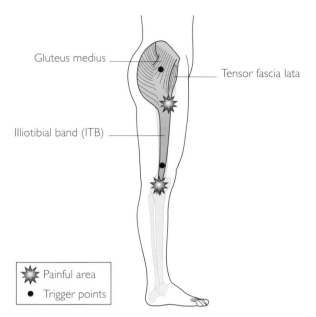

Figure 7.9 ITB friction areas

The management of this condition involves stretching the ITB if it is tight, and both correcting faulty movements (movement dysfunction) at the hip and improving hip stability. You can use two tests as a guide to your training requirements. The first measures the tightness of the ITB; the second, stability and control of the hip.

ITB ASSESSMENT

ITB tightness is assessed using a physiotherapy procedure called the *Ober test*. Lie on your side with the leg to be tested on top. Bend your knee to 90 degrees, keeping your thigh in line with your body. Lift your top leg upwards (abduction) and then backwards (extension) (*see* fig 7.10a). Keeping the extension (your leg should always be slightly behind the line of your body), lower your leg without allowing your pelvis to dip or your

spine to bend to the side (*see* fig 7.10b). Ideally you should be able to lower your leg at least to the horizontal, if not further. If your leg stops above the horizontal, your ITB is very tight and requires stretching. If it only just reaches the horizontal, you are borderline and would be well advised to use the ITB stretches within your training programme.

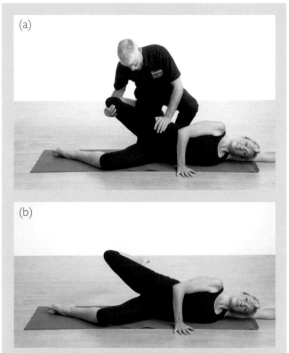

Figure 7.10 Ober test: (a) test position; (b) self stretch

Keypoint

The *Ober test* is used to measure flexibility of the ITB. It may also be adapted as a stretching exercise.

For the second test, stand on one leg in shorts and have your partner stand behind you. As you stand on one leg your pelvis (shown as the waistband of your shorts) should stay horizontal. This action is held by your powerful side hip muscles (gluteus medius and tensor fascia lata, or TFL), and if these are weak your pelvis will dip down (*see* figs 7.11a and 7.11b), indicating poor hip/pelvic stability. For the second part of this test, again stand on one leg. Now, gradually bend your knee. Your training partner should see your knee remain over your foot and not drift inwards (*see* fig 7.11c), again indicating poor stability. If your knee does drift inwards see if you can correct this by pressing it outwards and taking your bodyweight over the outside of your foot. If your knee drifts but you can correct it, your hip instability is through poor control; if you cannot correct it, your instability is through muscle weakness.

MASSAGE AND TRIGGER POINTS

ITB syndrome responds to self-massage aimed at lengthening fascia and eliminating trigger points. The ITB runs from the outside of your hip to the outside of your knee and can be most effectively reached by sitting on the floor with your legs crossed, keeping your uninjured leg straight and bending your injured leg to 90 degrees. From this position use the tips of your fingers grouped together or a specialised massage tool (*see* fig 4.14, page 54) to press into the ITB from the outer hip bone (greater trochanter) down to the knee.

Trigger points are painful local areas which often feel like small nodules or bands within tissue. Two trigger points are commonly found in the ITB: one high up on the hip between the front of the pelvic rim (iliac spine) and the outer hip bone, the other about two hand widths above the knee.

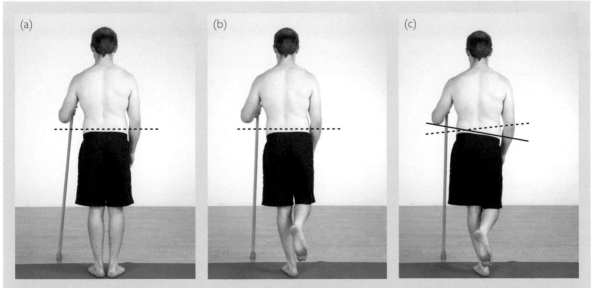

Figure 7.11 Hip dip test: (a) normal standing (b) single leg standing – the pelvis is level (c) single leg standing – the pelvis dips

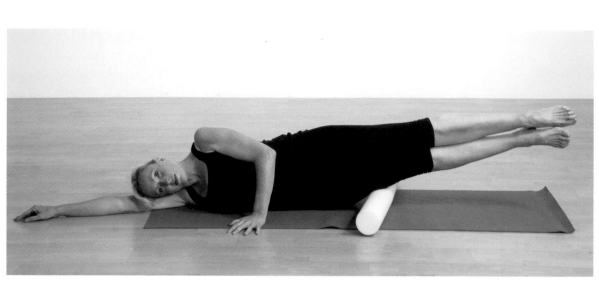

Figure 7.12 Trigger point release using a foam roller

The trigger points can be released using firm direct pressure. Lie on your side with a foam roller beneath your outer thigh. Move your body up and down until you position the roller over the most painful area – this is the trigger point location (*see* fig 7.12). Hold the position with the weight of your leg pushing down onto the roller for 20–30 seconds. Another effective way to release trigger points is to use a ball. Stand side on to a wall and place a ball between the wall and your leg. Press your leg against the wall to push the ball into the ITB at the most painful spot (*see* fig 7.13). Hold this position for 30–60 seconds and slowly release. You may need to vary the position of the ball and use the technique several times before the trigger point releases. As pain subsides in the trigger point apply the stretches detailed below.

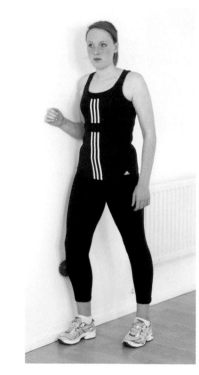

Figure 7.13 Trigger point release using a spiky ball

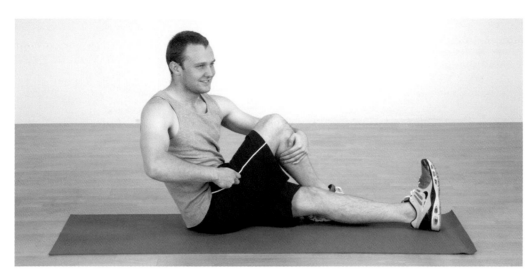

Figure 7.14 ITB stretch – sitting

EXERCISES

ITB stretch – sitting

Purpose
To lengthen the ITB focusing on the upper portion.

Preparation
Sit on the floor with your legs crossed. Keep your uninjured leg straight and bend your injured leg to 90 degrees.

Action
If the ITB is very tight and painful, maintain this stretched position until pain eases. Next, use your hand to press the knee of your bent leg over and down to the ground (*see* fig 7.14).

Tips
You can vary the stretch by lifting your foot off the ground and pulling your knee up towards your chest, keeping it in the crossed-over position.

ITB stretch – kneeling

Purpose
To stretch the whole length of the ITB.

Preparation
Begin kneeling on one knee (your painful side) on a folded towel or cushion.

Action
Press your pelvis forwards and then sideways towards your painful side. Hold this stretched position for 30 seconds and then slowly release.

Tips
This action presses your hip backwards (extension) and inwards (adduction). To feel an effective stretch it is important that you maintain good spinal alignment – do not allow your low back to hollow.

Hip hitch

Purpose
To strengthen the muscles feeding into the ITB.

Preparation
Stand facing a chair with your arms outstretched and fingers on the back of the chair for balance.

Action
Keeping your knees locked and legs straight, hitch one hip upwards so that your heel clears the floor by 5–10 cm (*see* fig 7.15b). Hold the upper position for 5 seconds and then rest. Repeat on the other leg, performing 5 reps on each side.

Tips
This action strengthens the outer hip muscles (gluteus medius and TFL), which can also be worked using the clamshell exercise (*see* fig 7.2) on page 96.

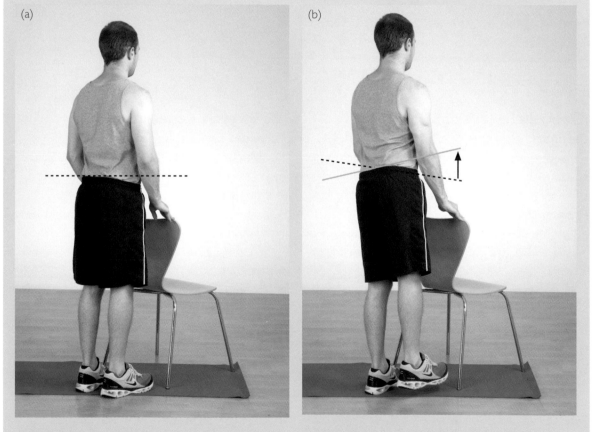

Figure 7.15 Hip hitch (a) start position (b) hitch one hip upwards

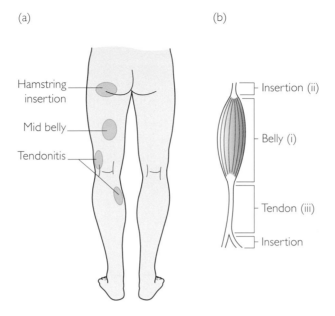

Figure 7.16 Hamstring injury: (a) site of pain (b) site of injury on muscle structure

HAMSTRING TEAR

The *hamstrings* are a group of three muscles stretching from your sitting bone to the back of your shinbone (tibia). A portion of one of your adductor muscles (the vertical fibres of adductor magnus) also travels with the hamstrings and is sometimes called the *4th hamstring*. The hamstrings have a special make-up because they work over both the knee and hip joints. The coordination involved with this action can sometimes break down and is an important feature of injury. This same coordination is important to work during rehabilitation because failure to do so can leave you open to re-injury.

Three types of hamstring injury are seen in sport: *mid-belly tear (i), hamstring insertion tear (ii) and hamstring tendonitis (iii)* (*see* fig 7.16). Mid-belly tearing is the most common type and gives pain in the middle of the back of the thigh.

This typically occurs through running. You may step onto some loose gravel and slip as you turn or lengthen your pace, or simply pull up when tired towards the end of a game. You feel a pain in the back of your thigh and with each step it gets worse as your leg stretches forwards.

Hamstring insertion tearing normally occurs with more force, and when you are lifting your trunk from your hips in actions such as a deadlift in the gym, pushing in a scrum, or performing a judo throw. You feel pain right up into your sitting bone, and an ache and often tingling travel into the back of your thigh. You find sitting uncomfortable, and straightening your leg gives tightness and pain up into your buttock.

Hamstring tendon pain (*tendinopathy*) is felt at the knee, either on the inside or on the outside. It normally occurs after endurance activities and may be mistaken for knee injury. As the tendons travel close to the knee there are small balloon-like structures called *bursas* which stop the tendons from rubbing over the bone. These can also become inflamed (bursitis) at the same time as the hamstring tendons. With this type of injury the intensity of training must be reduced, but any alignment fault to the knee or foot must also be identified, as these sometimes subtle changes, if missed, will mean that an injury comes back after the body part has been rested and training resumes.

Hamstring injury may coincide with pain from the sciatic nerve and the slump test is used by physiotherapists to differentiate the two (*see* chapter 8, page 122).

Keypoint
Pain which appears to be coming from a hamstring injury may be from the sciatic nerve. Physiotherapists use the slump test to distinguish between the two.

TAPING
Taping for a hamstring injury can be used to compress an area and reduce the spread of swelling; to unload the muscle (the tape takes some of the stress normally taken by the muscle); and to re-educate and guide the direction of a movement.

To *compress* an area after injury:

• Apply an underwrap or shave the skin and apply a protective spray (skin prep).

• Place elastic tape over the area, stretching each piece before it is attached to the skin. The strips

are placed across the muscle fibres that is perpendicular to the thigh (*see* fig 7.17).

• As the tape recoils when stuck to the skin it will tighten the skin and fascia over the area, restricting the spread of swelling and bleeding through the muscle.

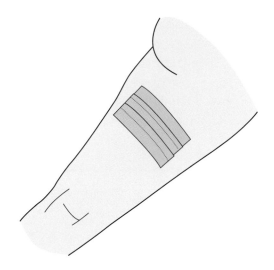

Figure 7.17 Elastic tape is placed on the hamstring and is used to change the underlying muscle tone

To *unload* the hamstrings and restrict movement:

• Use non-elastic tape to part or all of the muscle.

• Have your injured partner lie on their front and place a cushion under their shin to relax the hamstrings.

• Apply anchors above and below the painful areas. Next, attach strips of tape between the anchors along the length of the muscle.

- The muscle lies beneath the skin, and so applying taping in this way will not directly affect the muscle. However, any tightness of the tape on the skin will remind your partner not to stretch out fully, and make the area feel more supported. Nevertheless, taping should not be applied to allow them to compete on an injured muscle when further injury may be caused.

To *re-educate* movement:

- Use non-elastic tape placed directly on the skin. Taping has been shown to change the tone of a muscle and may be used to remind a player of an aspect of a movement.

- For example, if your partner is pressing a weight overhead (push press) when standing and you see their knee overextending, this can place stress on the hamstrings causing tendonitis.

- Placing tape on the back of the knee when it is slightly bent (X-tape) will remind them not to lock the knee out.

- If they try to do so the tape will tighten, pulling on their skin and giving them feedback.

MASSAGE

Massage to the hamstrings may be either *general* or *specific*. General massage aims to improve blood flow to the area, relax the muscle and ease pain. Specific massage focuses on local tissue mobilisation.

Ask your partner to lie down on their front with their knee bent. Place a cushion beneath their shin to relax the hamstrings. Use cream or oil as a massage lubricant and begin the massage using flat-hand stroking actions (effleurage) from the knee to the buttock. Gradually increase the depth of the movement and then change to picking up and kneading actions (*see* fig 7.18, page 112). For picking up, grasp the muscles using flat fingers (do not dig your fingertips into the skin) and draw the muscle upwards (*see* fig 7.18b, page 112). To knead the muscle, again draw the muscle up and then move your hands backwards and forwards relative to each other. Work your way up the whole length of the muscle. To stimulate the muscle circulation, use percussion techniques, striking the skin with your fingertips or the sides of the (open) hand (*see* fig 7.18c, page 112). Finish the massage by repeating your stroking actions.

Specific massage may be given using local pressure from your fingertips to break up swelling, or deep transverse frictions (DTF) across the muscle fibres. For DTF you should press firmly into the skin so that your fingers move with the skin, rather than across it.

EXERCISES

Active knee extension
Purpose
To encourage relaxation and stretch of the hamstrings using muscle reflexes.

Preparation
Lie on the floor and bend your injured leg, drawing your knee up above your hip.

Action
Cup your hands around the back of your thigh and straighten your leg using your quads power only (*see* fig 7.19, page 112). Hold the stretched position for 10–20 seconds and perform 3–5 reps.

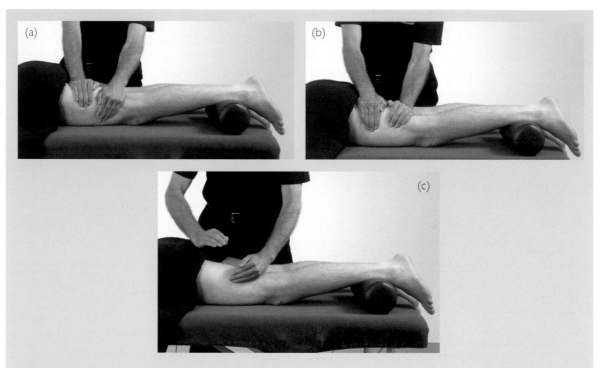

Figure 7.18 Massage techniques for the posterior thigh: (a) kneading (b) picking up (c) percussion

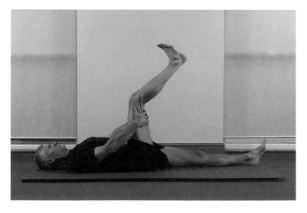

Figure 7.19 Active knee extension

Tips

You may not be able to straighten your leg completely to lock out your knee. This is fine, as the stretch is still effective. The exercise uses a PNF technique, where the muscle tone of the contracting quads causes the hamstrings to reduce their tone slightly, easing the stretch.

Hamstring upper insertion stretch
Purpose

To stretch the hamstrings focusing on the upper portion into the buttock.

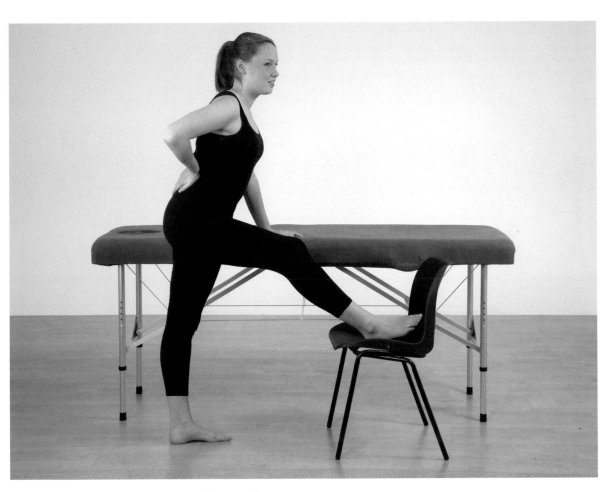

Figure 7.20 Hamstring upper insertion stretch

Preparation

Place a chair or gym bench close to a handhold for balance (high cupboard or gym machinery). Stand facing the chair and place your injured foot onto the chair seat, keeping your knee bent to 20–30 degrees.

Action

Keep your back straight and tip your trunk forwards, hinging from your hip. Your sitting bone should move backwards (anterior pelvic tilt) and you should feel the stretch up into your buttock (*see* fig 7.20).

Tips

This stretch is only effective if your spine stays still and your pelvis tilts. If you bend your back the stretch is taken from the hamstrings and placed on the low back instead.

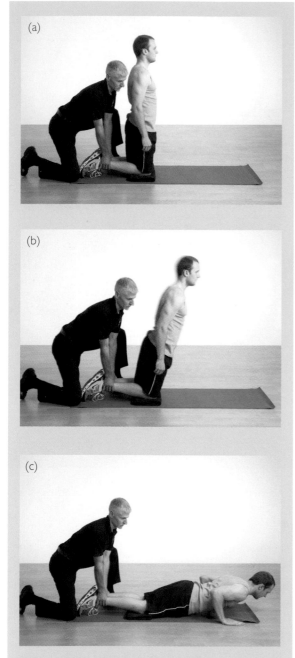

Figure 7.21 Nordic hamstring exercise: (a) start (b) mid position (c) finish position

Nordic hamstring exercise

Purpose

To strengthen the hamstrings while lengthening (eccentric contraction).

Preparation

Begin kneeling with your knees on a mat or two folded towels. Ask your training partner to hold your feet (*see* fig 7.21a).

Action

Keep your back straight and lower your body into the press-up position (*see* fig 7.21b and 7.21c). Use your hands to push yourself back up again and repeat for 10 reps.

Tips

This exercise can be made harder by slowing your descent. Begin by lowering in 1–2 seconds and build up to 5–10 seconds.

Straight leg deadlift

Purpose

To strengthen the hamstrings using a functional movement.

Preparation

Begin facing a light (5–10 kg) barbell placed at mid-shin level. Bend forwards, keeping your back straight, and angle your trunk forwards 45 degrees to grip the bar. Place your hands shoulder width apart.

Action

Keeping your back and legs straight, lift the bar by pulling your trunk back up to the vertical position (*see* fig 7.22, page 115).

Tips

If you find it difficult to perform this action, begin with the barbell higher (hip height), placed on two benches. The action is complex and may need close supervision from a personal trainer.

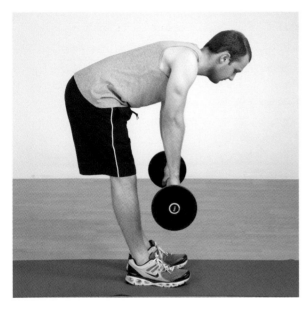

Figure 7.22 Straight leg deadlift

When you have stretched and strengthened and no longer have pain with any of the exercises, it is time to begin the return to sport by using running drills.

RUNNING DRILLS

You must use a progressive programme of running drills, rather than simply moving from controlled gym-based exercise to rapid running. Table 7.1 (overleaf) shows an example progression. Use the running drills every other day so that you have a day's rest for your muscles to recover. When you can perform a drill comfortably without any pain you can progress to the next one. You do not have to use each drill – pick the ones which suit your injury and sport. The drills address hamstring, groin, quads and knee rehab requirements.

Terms you should know:

Impingement – compression of tissue through pinching between two body structures.

Ober test – a measure of flexibility of the illiotibial band (ITB).

PNF – standing for *proprioceptive neuromuscular facilitation*, this is a type of stretching that utilises muscle reflexes to improve the stretching effect.

Tendinopathy – any painful condition affected tendons. This may be through inflammation, damage or incorrect healing.

Trigger point – a hypersensitive nodular area within a muscle. Often the cause of pain which may travel (refer) for some distance.

Table 7.1 Running drills

Drills	Coaching points
Speed walking	Begin slowly and build up speed. Focus on a correct walking style (gait pattern). Make sure that your feet are parallel (don't turn them out) and each step (stride) is of equal length. Listen to the sound of your feet striking the ground – they should sound the same. If not, your stride pattern is different on one side of your body.
Scouts pace	Walk 10 paces and then jog 5 paces. Repeat this for 2–5 minutes and then walk 10 paces and jog 10 paces. Build up until you are jogging for 20 to 30 paces and walking for 10.
Cross jogging	Begin jogging with small, even strides. Lengthen your strides, then shorten them. Perform some jogging on road and some off road, some on the flat and some on hills. Create as much variety as you can, gradually increasing the time and intensity of your run.
Side step	Face sideways and side step at a jogging pace. Perform 10–15 steps leading with your right leg and then the same number leading with your left.
Walking lunge	Stand with your feet hip width apart. Step forwards (one leg length) with your right foot and bend your right knee to 90 degrees, allowing your left knee to bend and touch the ground lightly. Now, step forwards with your left. Move forwards at a walking pace for 10 steps and then rest. Ensure that your knee passes over your foot – do not allow your knee to drift inwards.
Carioca	Face sideways with your feet apart. Step behind your right leg with your left, then step sideways with your right and finally step in front of your right leg with your left. Continue this rhythm of front-side-behind for 10–20 paces.
Running backwards	Running backwards works your hamstrings and gluteal muscles more and is excellent for balance. Make sure your path is clear to avoid tripping.
Zigzag running	Set up 8–10 markers (cones). Begin jogging towards them and move to the sides, working your way between them. Your action can be a powerful side lunge rather than several small paces.
Lengthening pace	Begin jogging and then stride out for 10 paces. Come back to jogging to recover before striding once again.
Sprint from mark	Jog for 2–3 minutes and then stop and stand still. Sprint for 10 paces and jog to recover.
Clock face lunge	Stand in the centre of a large space and place markers at 12 o'clock, 6 o'clock, 9 o'clock and 3 o'clock. Ask your training partner to call out the time and you should lunge to reach that point. Return to the centre point each time before lunging once again.
Hurdle jump	Stand on one side of a rope or low hurdle. Jump over the hurdle, keeping your feet slightly apart. Jump forwards and backwards, and then side to side.
Harness run	Place a webbing belt or commercial harness around your waist. Ask your training partner to hold the harness and run forwards as they try to slow you down by pulling backwards. You should dig your feet into the ground and pump your arms hard as you power forwards with your legs.
Tyre pull	Attach a tyre to your harness and run forwards against its resistance.

LOW BACK

8

Low back pain (LBP) affects four out of five people, and unfortunately sports people are not immune from this condition. However, exercise is an effective treatment for LBP providing it is applied correctly. Let's begin with a brief overview of the structures of the low back. For more in depth information see chapter 1 'How the Spine Works' in *Abdominal Training* (3rd edition) by Christopher Norris published by A&C Black (2009).

Each spinal bone (vertebra) has three joints. In the centre is the *spinal disc*. This is a little like a toothpaste tube in that it has a gel centre (nucleus) and a hard outer casing (annulus) (*see* fig 8.1). Acting as a shock absorber as you move, the disc will bend and change shape as the spinal bones change their alignment to each other. Squeezing the disc pressurises its gel, making it firmer to offer greater support. Too much pressure, however, can cause the gel to slowly ooze, or rapidly burst, through its outer casing, causing severe injury.

On either side of the disc are two smaller joints called *facets*. These are similar in construction to your knee or elbow in that they are synovial joints

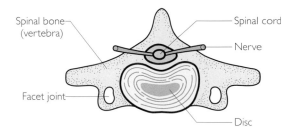

Figure 8.1 Cross-section through the spine

containing joint fluid and have a capsule and ligaments. These structures are susceptible to the same injuries as any other joint, such as joint locking, tissue becoming trapped, ligament spraining and joint swelling.

The whole spine is strengthened by two sets of muscles: those which travel from joint to joint (*unisegmental*) and those travelling the whole length of the spine (*multisegmental*). However, the spine has an important further support mechanism and that is *core stability*, which we will cover in this chapter. Let's first turn our attention to perhaps the most severe type of injury, that of the disc.

Keypoint

The spine is covered by two sets of muscles. General muscles running the full length of the spine (multisegmental) and local muscles running only between two adjacent spinal bones (unisegmental).

SLIPPED DISC

The spinal disc functions a little like a toothpaste tube (disc) between two bricks (vertebrae). The disc is under pressure, and as we carry things the pressure is increased and the disc is squeezed down. In fact after 25 minutes of weight training the disc shrinks in height by over 5 mm. In addition to this vertical pressure, the disc is pressed out of shape as we bend. The vertebrae alter their alignment to each other, a little like the bricks tilting, and so the disc is squeezed at the front and stretched at the back. These squeezing and pressing movements are not normally a problem as the disc was designed to be active. However, our day-to-day lives can put an excessive amount of one type of stress on the disc through continually sitting at desks and in cars, and this combined with obesity, poor diet and lack of exercise can leave the disc tissue in poor shape. When this happens a sudden excessive force (normally bending forwards and twisting) can cause the disc gel to burst through the disc casing, giving a slipped (prolapsed) disc (*see* fig 8.2, page 119). On X-ray the spinal bones are seen to be closer together (loss of disc height), and if the disc gel presses on a nerve, the condition is extremely painful. Because nerves carry impulses for both feeling (sensory) and moving (motor), both of these functions can be affected by disc injury. You may get pain in the back or down your leg where the nerve runs. In addition, muscles which are supplied by the nerve will be weak. The nerve in question is called the *sciatic nerve*, and so the condition is called *sciatica*.

Keypoint

A slipped (or prolapsed) disc occurs when the central gel of the disc bursts through the outer disc casing.

MECHANICAL THERAPY

One of the most effective ways to combat a disc injury is an exercise programme designed to alter pressure within the disc and squeeze it back into shape. The exercises form part of a physiotherapy approach called *mechanical therapy* (the McKenzie programme). The key point about these exercises is that they involve repeated actions to have a pumping effect on the disc. When this happens, the pain centralises. This means that it starts to shrink back to where it came from. If you have a disc injury which gives you pain down to your knee, after performing McKenzie exercises the pain would just go into your buttock to begin with, and after performing the exercises a little longer, the pain appears just in your back. This shows that pressure within the back is changing mechanically. Importantly, if this does not occur and the pain stays where it is, travels further down the leg or gets worse, you should see a physiotherapist straight away as your disc pain may be more complicated.

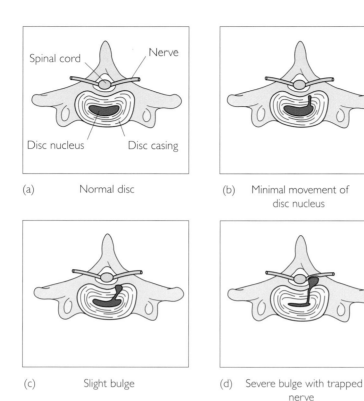

(a)   Normal disc

(b)   Minimal movement of disc nucleus

(c)   Slight bulge

(d)   Severe bulge with trapped nerve

Figure 8.2 The spinal disc and injury

Keypoint

When performing McKenzie exercises your pain should centralise. If it does not, stop the exercises and see a physiotherapist immediately.

EXERCISES

Side gliding – standing

Purpose

To correct a side bend (shift) posture resulting from back pain.

Preparation

Begin standing side on to a wall with your painful side away from the wall. Place your forearm on the wall at shoulder height.

Action

Gently press your hips in towards the wall without shrugging your shoulders (*see* fig 8.3, overleaf). Perform 10 reps of the movement rhythmically. Rest and repeat until your posture is straighter and your pain has moved higher up your leg (centralised).

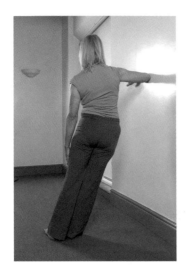

Figure 8.3 Side gliding – standing

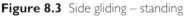

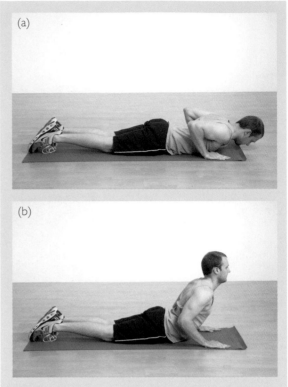

Figure 8.4 Low back extension – lying: (a) start position (b) mid position

Tips

Normally if you have pain on the right side of your back you will tend to lean sideways away from the pain (left shift). In this case you begin the exercise with your left shoulder against the wall. If your pain does not change, rest and repeat the exercise with your right arm against the wall.

Low back extension – lying

Purpose

To restore the natural curve to the low back (lumbar lordosis) and centralise back pain.

Preparation

Begin lying on the floor with your arms bent and hands flat on the floor by your shoulders (press-up position) (*see* fig 8.4a).

Action

Keeping your hips on the floor, press with your arms to bend your spine (*see* fig 8.4b). Go up as high as is comfortable and perform 10 reps rhythmically. Rest and repeat, gradually increasing the distance you are able to raise your body.

Tips

There is a tendency for the hips to lift, which takes the work off the low back and makes the exercise less effective. Have your training partner press into the small of your back (just above the waistband of your trousers) to keep your hips down.

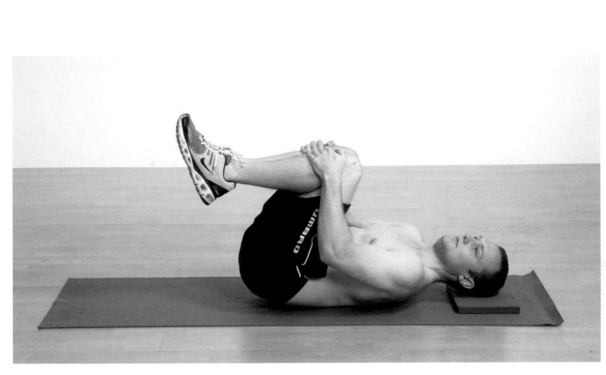

Figure 8.5 Low back flexion – lying

Low back flexion – lying

Purpose

To mobilise the low back and reduce the lumbar curve where it is excessive.

Preparation

Begin lying on the floor. Draw your knee up towards your chest, lifting them one at a time. Cup your hands around your knees.

Action

Pull your knees up and in, aiming your kneecaps towards your upper chest (*see* fig 8.5). Your tailbone should raise off the floor slightly, but your mid back (thoracic spine) should stay supported on the floor. Perform 5–10 reps.

Tips

As you lower your knees back to the floor at the end of the exercise, do so one at a time, keeping them bent. Lowering both legs together or keeping them straight can place excessive stress on your back.

NEURAL TENSION

Following an injury where your nerve has been trapped or swelling has spread onto it, the nerve itself may be tight. Nerves are contained within a sheath, a little like a bicycle brake cable. As you bend and straighten, the nerve should slide up and down unhindered. If swelling sticks to the nerve sheath as healing progresses, the sliding of the nerve can be affected causing pain. We call this *neural tension* and it can occur in the leg following LBP or in the arm following neck pain (whiplash, for example). You get pain in the leg or arm, and sometimes the pain may just be in one spot. For example, after you have started to recover from LBP you may notice that you get tingling (pins and needles) or numbness in your foot when driving. The driving position actually gives us guidance as to a test for this condition, called the *slump test*.

SLUMP TEST

The slump test tries to tension each part of the neural system in turn, tightening the nerves in the spine, leg and arms. Each is then released to discover where the tension lies.

To begin the slump sit on a high bench or table. Link your hands behind you and bend your whole spine as though trying to put your nose onto your stomach. Straighten your unaffected leg and pull your toes towards you. This will feel tight and slightly achy. Lower this leg and then straighten your painful leg again, pulling your toes towards you. This should create your pain (or tingling). To confirm that neural tension is the cause of the pain, keep your leg exactly as it is but look up and straighten your spine without moving your pelvis. If the pain eases off, the cause is tension in the neural system (nerves and spinal cord), rather than your leg itself being injured. This is because the pain has eased even though the leg, hip and pelvic position has not been altered. A positive slump test means that nerve stretching is required, and we begin by using the slump test as an exercise.

Keypoint

The slump test combines movement of the leg, spine, neck and arm.

Slump stretch
Purpose
To mobilise the neural system focusing on the leg.

Preparation
Begin sitting on a high bench or table. Link your hands behind you and bend your whole spine as though trying to put your nose onto your stomach.

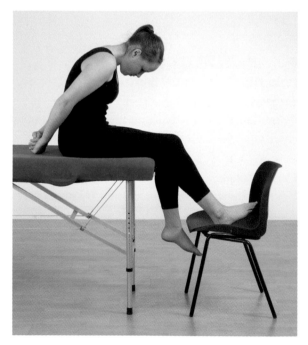

Figure 8.6 Slump stretch

Action

Slowly straighten your painful leg, pointing your toes away from you (plantar flexion). Hold this position for 5 seconds and then if not too painful pull your toes towards you (dorsiflexion). Hold for a further 5 seconds and then release. Release your arms, allow your legs to bend and sit up straight to recover. Repeat the slump stretch for 3 reps.

Tips

Nerves are very delicate so it is important to apply the stretch gradually. The feeling should be intense but not painful (2 or 3 out of 10 on a pain scale, but no higher). As you release the stretch your heel should rest on the floor. If your table is too high for this, place your heel on a chair and perform the stretch from this level (*see* fig 8.6, page 122).

Forward bend – sitting

Purpose

To mobilise the neural tissue giving overpressure to the foot and calf.

Preparation

Begin sitting on the floor. Grasp a towel with both hands and place it around your feet (forefoot level).

Action

Keep your knees locked and pull on the towel to draw your feet towards you. At the same time bend your trunk forwards, aiming your forehead to your knees (*see* fig 8.7). Hold the stretch for 3–5 seconds and then release. Repeat for 3–5 reps.

Tips

This is an intense nerve stretch and you should ease into the movement and not force it. Normally with a forward bend you should aim to maintain good spinal alignment by keeping your spine straight, but this stretch deliberately bends (flexes) the spine to target the neural system. It must be performed gently to guard against back injury.

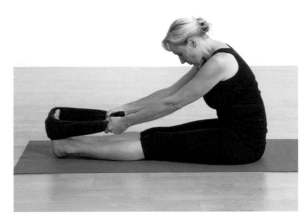

Figure 8.7 Forward bend – sitting

BACK MUSCLE PAIN

Back pain does not necessarily have to involve the discs, nerves or lumbar joints. Pain may simply come from muscle tension and spasm. The two main muscles are the pair of thick spinal extensors on either side of the spine (erector spinae) and the QL (quadratus lumborum), which are deep side flexor muscles running from the back rim of the pelvis to the lower ribs. You will feel the muscles hard and painful and they will limit movement. In the case of the spinal extensors you will find it difficult to bend forwards or to the sides as though your back were 'locked'. When the QL is tight the pain is deep into the back on one side and you find it difficult to bend to one side but not the other.

With this type of back pain you can use massage to release tension and trigger points, heat or ice to reduce pain, and exercise to stretch out tight muscles and correct movement dysfunction. Often it is the combination of these techniques that is most effective.

MASSAGE, HEAT AND ICE

Heat is very soothing on back spasm, and a hot shower or hot water bottle is often your first line of defence at home. Microwavable hot packs will penetrate slightly deeper as they give moist heat, which soaks into the skin. An infrared heat lamp will warm a larger area and leave the skin red (erythema), showing an increase in skin blood flow. Similar changes to the skin can be brought about by applying ice or giving ice massage along the spinal extensors which can be used to relieve severe spasm. One word of caution, however; tight muscle may be in protective spasm. In this case the spasm is protecting an underlying injury or medical condition. If the pain and spasm do not begin to reduce within a few days you should see your physiotherapist to have a full spinal assessment.

Massage is performed with your partner lying on their front. It is often more comfortable to put a pillow or soft cushion under the abdomen to lessen the deep spinal curve (lordosis). Begin using long stroking actions (effleurage), pointing your fingertips towards the head (*see* fig 8.8a). Press

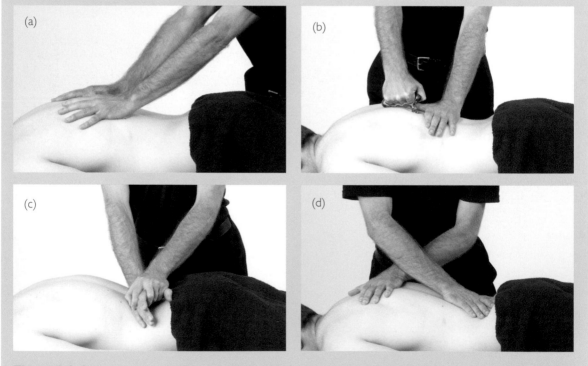

Figure 8.8 Back massage: (a) effleurage (b) local pressure using a massage tool (c) local pressure using the heel of the hand (d) fascial stretch using X-grip

Keypoint
Back muscles may be in protective spasm, disguising an underlying medical condition. If pain does not begin to ease within a couple of days see your physiotherapist for a full spinal assessment.

firmly over the low back but ease off as you get to the ribcage. Use pressure from one hand supported by the other to provide deep sideways (lateral) pressure, and focus on local painful areas using your fingertips or a massage tool (*see* fig 8.8b, page 124). Stretch the skin and fascia using strong pressure with an X-grip (*see* fig 8.8d, page 124). If you are standing on the left side of your partner, put your right hand on their mid back and your left on their low back so your arms cross. Lean forwards, pressing on your hands so that they spread apart and stretch the skin. The QL is often more effectively treated with your partner lying on their side over a folded pillow. Press gently into the pain area between the pelvis and lower ribs.

EXERCISES

Spinal rotation on a chair
Purpose
To place overpressure on spinal rotation and ensure rotation symmetry.

Preparation
Begin sitting side on to a firm chair. Sit upright with your knees and hips at 90 degrees. Turn towards the chair back and grasp the back at each side with both hands (*see* fig 8.9).

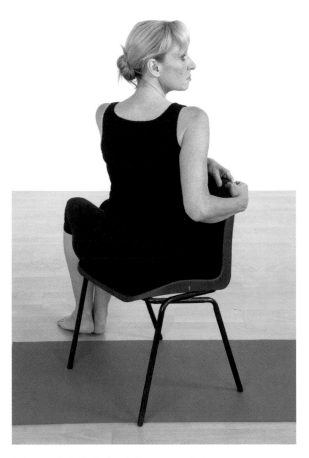

Figure 8.9 Spinal rotation on a chair

Action
Inhale and as you exhale turn your spine further towards the chair back while pulling with your arms to encourage further movement. Release and allow your spine to rotate back to the starting position. Perform 5 reps and then turn (180 degrees) to sit facing the other side and repeat.

Tips
The action should be gentle overpressure to encourage movement, but not aggressive pulling

to force it. It is common for one side of the body to be stiffer than the other. Concentrate on the stiffer side, trying to make both sides equal (symmetrical).

Flexion – standing

Purpose

To stretch the spinal extensor muscles.

Preparation

Begin standing with one foot resting on a chair seat.

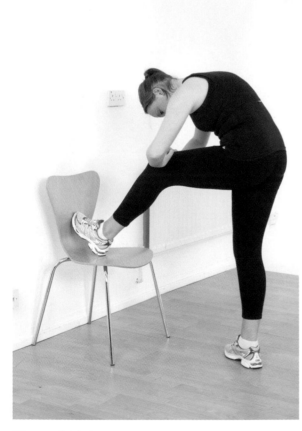

Figure 8.10 Flexion – standing

Action

Grasp your thigh and bend (flex) your spine as though trying to touch your knee with your head (*see* fig 8.10). Gently pull with your hands to encourage further movement.

Tips

This exercise is designed to increase bending of the back (spinal flexion) so the action is to pull your head towards your knee. The same position may be used to stretch the hamstring muscles, where the aim would be to maintain good spinal alignment and keep your spine straight.

Supported side flexion

Purpose

To lengthen the trunk side flexors and open the spinal joints on one side.

Preparation

Begin standing side on to a table or bench. Rest your closest arm on the table and reach your furthest arm overhead.

Action

Side bend towards the table, taking your bodyweight through your arm onto the table top. Reach your furthest arm over the top of the table, keeping it level with your ear. Hold the fully stretched position for 10 seconds and then move back to the starting position. Perform 3–5 reps and then turn around (180 degrees) to perform the exercise on the other side of your body (*see* fig 8.11, page 127).

Tips

The action should be pure side bending without twisting your spine. Imagine your body is

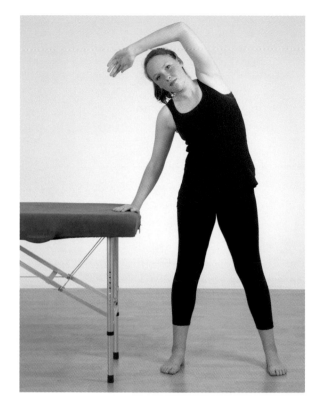

Figure 8.11 Supported side flexion

sandwiched between two sheets of glass so you cannot bend forwards and backwards or twist – you can only move sideways.

POSTURE IN SPORT

Posture has an important role to play in terms of back pain. Poor posture is a risk factor for the development of low back pain, but equally after a back injury individuals are often left with postural changes. Let's take a look at an optimal posture, changes which occur from this ideal, and examples of postural exercises which may be useful to restore correct postural alignment.

Good posture is all about balance. Viewed from the side your body should align along a vertical

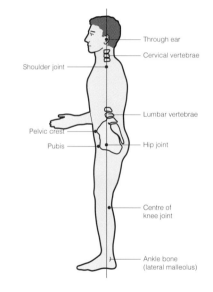

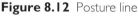

Figure 8.12 Posture line

posture line (*see* fig 8.12), with your ankle bone (lateral malleolus) on the line. The line should then pass through your knee joint, your hip joint, your shoulder joint and the centre of your ear. From the side the posture line passes down the centre of your spine and each part of your body should be equidistant from this line. Your knee creases, buttock creases, pelvis, shoulder blades and ears should all be at the same horizontal level and each should be the same distance from the central posture line. Table 8.1 gives you a checklist when comparing one side of your body to the other.

Where you discover postural changes from the optimal or ideal posture, these will often coincide with tissue changes that can be targeted with posture exercise. If one shoulder is higher than the other, for example, the shoulder muscles on the higher side will often be tight, requiring stretching. When your shoulders are rounded the muscles on

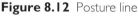

Table 8.1	**Checklist for assessing standing posture from behind**		
Part of the body	**Changes**	**Part of the body**	**Changes**
Ear level/hair line		Skin creases	
Shoulder level – cervical spine		Levels of pelvic rim, ASIS, belt line	
Inferior angle of scapula		Buttock creases	
Overall spinal alignment		Knee creases/ Muscle bulk	
Keyhole		Mid-line/ Achilles angle	
Adam's position		Foot position	

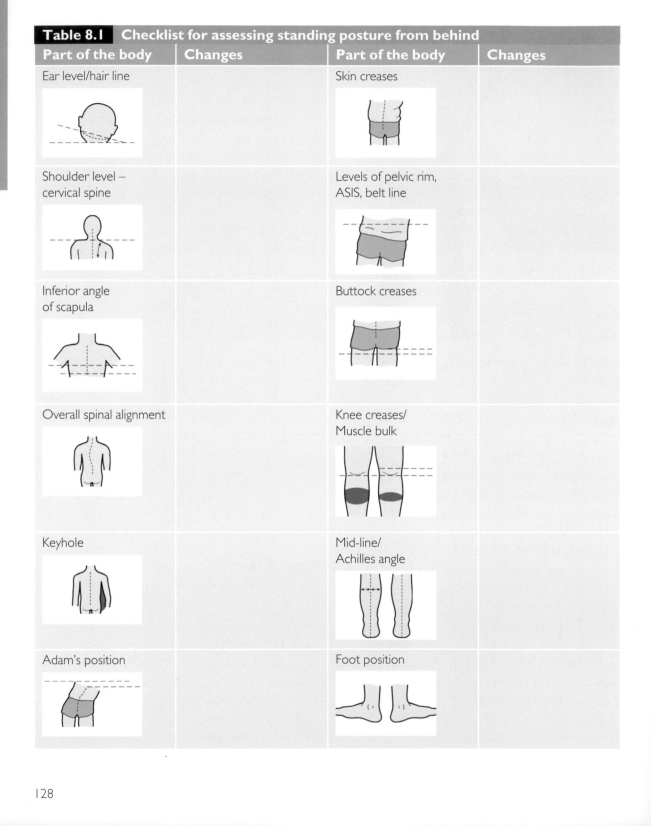

the back of your shoulder (shoulder retractors) are often lax, requiring strengthening.

Full postural correction is a specialist treatment requiring a full assessment and intervention from a physiotherapist, but there is a lot you can do for yourself at home or in the gym. One of the most important concepts with postural re-education is that of *mirror image exercise*. Here, we use the principle that repeated movement can often given rise to postural changes. We spend a lot of time sitting at desks, in front of computers and driving, for example. These are all bending (flexion) actions and so we end up with a bent forwards (round back) posture. To correct this we use exercises which move the body backwards (extension). Similarly, you may develop a postural change where one shoulder is stronger or higher than the other from single-handed sports or simply from carrying a computer bag with one hand. The postural change (muscular asymmetry) which has occurred is the result of over-strong and short muscles on one side of the body. This can be corrected by stretching the short muscles and strengthening the same muscles on the opposite side of the body to bring them up to the same level of strength and restore postural balance.

Table 8.2 shows examples of mirror image exercises for some common postural changes associated with back pain.

CORE STABILITY

Following any back injury your trunk muscles will have become weaker. To re-strengthen the muscles functionally you should use *core stability*. Functional training reflects the day-to-day usage of a body part, working many different muscles at the same time, whereas non-functional training generally uses one or two muscles in isolation.

> **Keypoint**
>
> Functional training reflects the day-to-day usage of a body part.

Muscle isolation can be important early on in rehabilitation, but functional exercise has the edge (*see* chapter 3) later on. In the case of the trunk, a sit-up exercise works the central abdominal muscle (rectus abdominis) particularly. The muscle is worked repeatedly to bend the spine.

However, this is not an action that we do repeatedly throughout the day. We may bend the spine to sit up from a lying position when we get up in the morning, but other than that we rarely use the action. Throughout the day you will lift, carry, push and pull objects. When you do this your arm and leg muscles are creating the movement, while your trunk muscles are protecting your spine from injury by holding it supported and firm.

The action of support rather than movement is what we refer to as *core stability*. This type of action mimics the day-to-day usage of the spine, and we will use a number of examples.

> **Definition**
>
> *Core stability* is functional exercise which mimics the support and protection given to the spine by the trunk muscles.

Table 8.2 Examples of postural therapy using mirror image exercises

Posture type	Exercise
Flat back 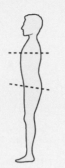 Curve in low back (lordosis) is reduced. Back is in **flexion**	**Low back extension stretch** 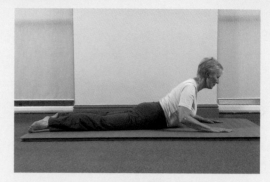 Encourage low back **extension** to increase low back curve
Round shoulder 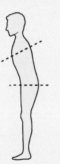 Chest muscles are tight and shoulders are **protracted**	**Chest stretch in corner of room** 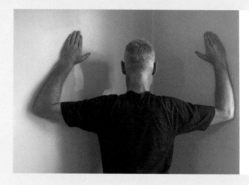 Lengthen chest muscles and **retract** shoulders
Hollow back 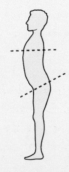 Abdominal muscles are lax and low back curve is increased. Back is in **extension**	**Low back flexion stretch** 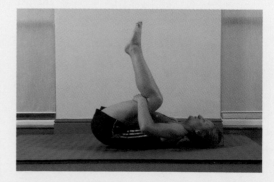 Encourage back **flexion**

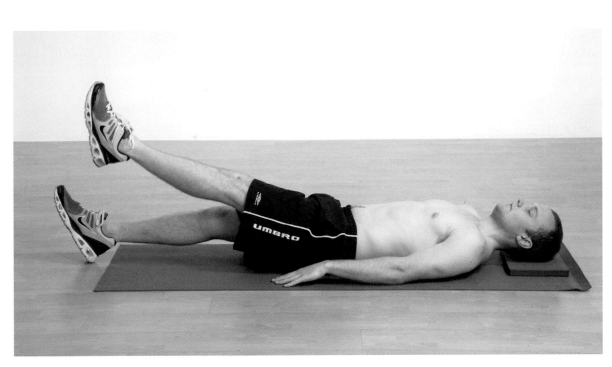

Figure 8.13 Single leg lift

EXERCISES

Single leg lift

Purpose
To activate the core stabilising muscles while moving the limbs.

Preparation
Lie on the floor with your legs straight. Adjust your spinal alignment so that the curve in the low back is normal (neutral position).

Action
Lift one leg to 30 degrees then lower it, lift the other leg and then lower (*see* fig 8.13). Repeat for 10–15 reps, maintaining the neutral position of your back – do not allow it to lift right off the floor.

Tips
This exercise begins with your low back in a *neutral position*. In this position your low back should not be flat against the floor (lumbar flexion) or overly arched away from it (lumbar extension). The neutral position is midway between the two extremes. You should be able to put one flat hand between your back and the floor. If you cannot get your hand into the space your back is too flat, and if you can get your whole fist in the space your back is too arched.

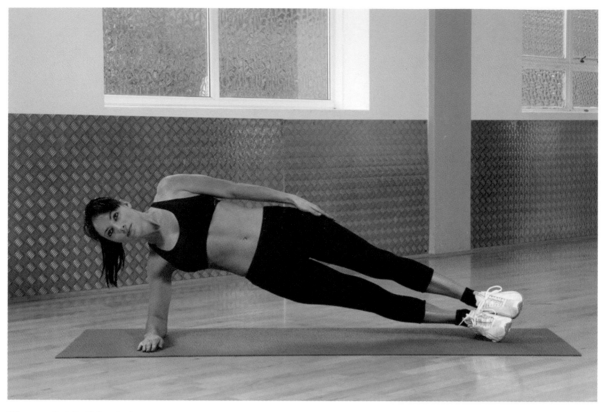

Figure 8.14 Side plank

Side plank

Purpose

To increase overload on the core stability muscles.

Preparation

Lie on your side with the sides of your feet on the floor, your top leg slightly in front of your bottom leg. Prop yourself up on your lower forearm.

Action

Straighten your body to lift your hips and knees from the floor. Your body should form a line from your feet to your shoulders, with your spine perfectly straight (*see* fig 8.14).

Tips

As you lift onto your underside arm, do not allow your shoulder to shrug. Maintain the distance between your ear and shoulder.

Deadlift

Purpose

To strengthen the legs, back and shoulders in a functional lifting action.

Preparation

Begin standing with your feet slightly apart, knees bent and shins touching a barbell positioned just below knee height. Grip the barbell with your hands shoulder width apart and to the sides of your knees. Lower your hips and straighten your back (*see* fig 8.15a).

Action

In a single movement straighten your legs and lift your trunk back up to the vertical position (*see* fig 8.15b). Pull the barbell close in towards you at all times.

Tips

If you find the action difficult to control, begin with the barbell resting on two stools so that it lies above rather than below your knees.

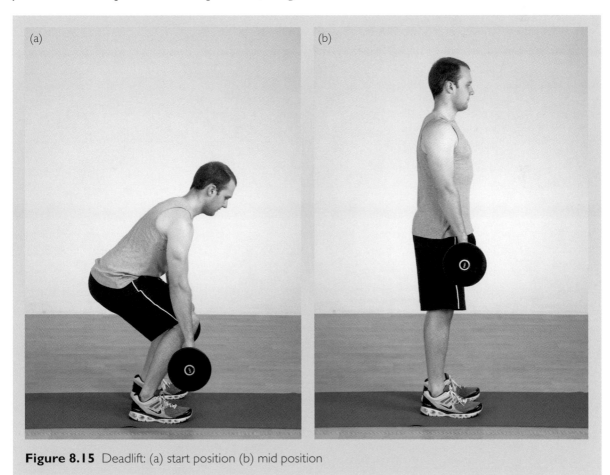

Figure 8.15 Deadlift: (a) start position (b) mid position

Walking lunge – arms overhead

Purpose
To maintain core stability while working the legs.

Preparation
Ensure that you can perform the lunge exercise (*see* chapter 6, page 90) for 10 reps before attempting this exercise. Begin holding a weight disc or single dumbbell (3–10 kg) above your head with arms locked out straight (*see* fig 8.16a).

Action
Step forwards with your right leg and bend your knees into the lunge position, aiming to get 90 degrees at both your knee and hip (*see* fig 8.16b). Press back up and then lunge with your left leg forwards (*see* fig 8.16c). Perform 10 steps in total, maintaining good spinal alignment throughout.

Tips
Make sure you perform single steps, getting your balance at the end of each step before performing the next. Once you have mastered this exercise you can perform the walking lunge backwards as well.

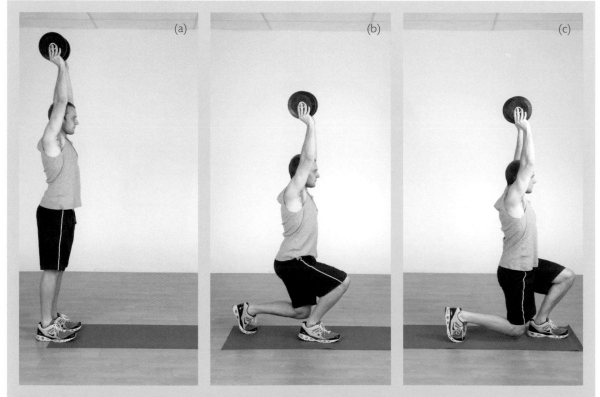

Figure 8.16 Walking lunge – arms overhead: (a) start position (b) step forwards with the right leg, bending into the lunge position (c) lunge with the left leg forwards

Terms you should know:

Core stability exercise – exercise which improves the support and protection given to the spine by the trunk muscles.

Facets – small flat joints lying either side of the spinal disc.

Mechanical therapy (the McKenzie programme) – a spinal therapy which involves rhythmical repeated movements.

Mirror image exercise – exercise which uses a movement opposite to that which caused a particular postural change.

Multisegmental muscle – muscle running across the whole length of the spine.

Neural tension – tightness in a nerve.

Prolapsed disc – the central gel of a disc bursting through the outer disc casing.

Slump test – a physiotherapy test which determines if nerve tightness is a component of a person's painful condition.

Unisegmental muscle – muscle running only between two neighbouring spinal bones (vertebrae).

RIBCAGE
// AND NECK

9

Many of the muscles working over the neck connect to the ribcage, and the ribs themselves connect to the thoracic (mid) spine. For this reason we will look at the two areas together. Both the *trapezius* muscle at the top of the shoulder and the *sternomastoid* muscle at the side of the neck connect to both the neck and shoulder. When they are tight your posture changes, raising one shoulder in a shrugging action and both tilting (lateral flexion) and twisting (rotating) the neck to one side. Postural evaluation is therefore vital when treating neck and ribcage injuries.

RIB JOINTS

The ribs connect to the thoracic spine at the back and the breastbone (sternum) at the front. Anything to do with the ribs is called *costo* in medical terms, so the joint with the sternum is the *sternocostal* (SC) joint, that with the vertebra the *costovertebral* (CV) joint and that with the side bone (transverse process) of the vertebra the *costotransverse* (CT) joint (*see* fig 9.1, page 137). Any of these joints may be injured through a kick in martial arts, a knee in rugby, or a fall (direct trauma). They may also inflame through poor technique in weight training exercise (overuse). Pain is generally felt over the immediate area

tracking along the rib. Pain increases as you take a deep breath because the ribs move on the rib joints. Trunk twist and side bend actions are also painful as the ribs slide and open up on the convex side (side away from the direction of bend). Sometimes the rib joints may partially dislocate (sublux), giving intense local pain which may resolve with a dull pop or thud as you stretch.

Rib injuries require a full assessment to ensure that no rib fracture is present. This typically gives intense pain to gentle pressure from the palm of the hand. Dull pain and the ability to move more easily suggests less severe rib injury, but your physiotherapist will be able to give a fuller picture. The area may be taped to make it more comfortable.

- Place elastic taping pre-stretched along or across the ribs in two or three overlapping pieces (*see* fig 9.2, page 137).

- Each tape strip is about 30 cm long and so does not surround the chest.

- The tape should support the chest without restricting breathing.

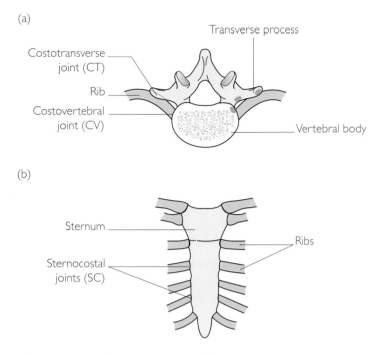

Figure 9.1 Rib joints: (a) with spine (b) with breastbone (sternum)

- Keep the tape on for no more than 2–3 days and then begin gentle exercise.

INTERCOSTAL MUSCLES

The *intercostal muscles* (there are three sets arranged in layers) lie between each adjacent pair of ribs and assist in breathing, and raising and lowering the ribs. They may be injured at the same time as the rib bones, or in isolation. Again, direct trauma or overuse involving rotation such as a repeated throwing action is normally the cause. They may also be injured during a bout of severe coughing.

Taping applied to the ribs will unload the intercostal muscles, and exercise can be used to regain their function. Massage between the ribs and individual rib joint mobilisation is also of use.

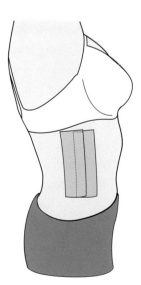

Figure 9.2 Rib taping – overlapping the tape by 50% strengthens the taping.

Massage between the ribs is best given with your partner lying on their side over a rolled towel or pillow. This position opens the ribs, exposing the intercostal muscles to your fingers. Massage along the length of the rib space using your fingertips (*see* fig 9.3a). Next, use a mobilisation to stretch the intercostal muscles. Use your fingertips or the side of your hand (*see* fig 9.3b) to hold down the rib below the level of injury. Maintaining this pressure, ask your partner to take a deep breath. This will lift the rib above your fingers and open the rib space. Further stretch may be given by holding the rib down and asking your partner to side bend slightly or rotate away from your hand. Choose the movement which your partner feels stretches the area most.

Having stretched the area, encourage your partner to breathe deeply, expanding the whole ribcage. Note that the breathing action involves four components: (i) *diagrammatic* (belly) breathing, where the abdominal wall expands outwards; (ii) *costal* breathing, where the lower ribs flare out; (iii) *sternal* breathing, where the breastbone lifts; and (iv) *apical* breathing, where the top ribs and collar bone (clavicle) lift upwards. Encourage your partner to feel air coming into the lungs (air entry) from the base to the sides, front and finally top as breathing goes through the sequence (i) to (iv). Where one of the components is poor, spend time focusing on this action and then progress to the exercises below.

EXERCISES

Deep breathing
Purpose
To maintain ribcage expansion and move the rib joints.

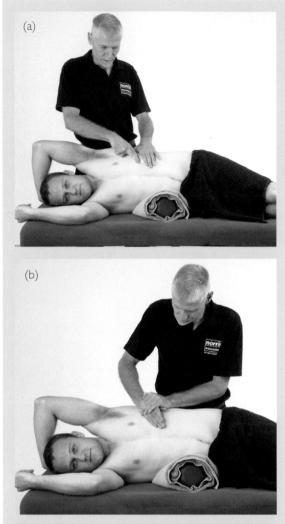

Figure 9.3 Intercostal massage: (a) massage along the length of the rib space (b) use a mobilisation technique

Preparation
Stand in front of a mirror with your ribcage exposed.

Action
Take a deep breath, making sure you expand the ribs at the bottom, then sides and finally top.

Keypoint

There are four components to the breathing action: *diagrammatic* (belly), *costal* (lower ribs), *sternal* (breastbone) and *apical* (collar bone) movements should all be detected.

Breathe as deeply as possible to expand your ribcage fully and hold the in breath (inspiration) for 5 seconds. Release and then breathe normally for 20–30 seconds before repeating. Perform 5 reps.

Tips

This exercise focuses on breathing in to expand the ribcage. To emphasise breathing out (expiration), blow into a balloon or use a commercially available breathing exerciser.

Deep breathing with arms raised

Purpose

To expand the ribcage and place overpressure on chest stretching.

Preparation

Sit on a bench or firm chair and grip a stick (broom handle) with each hand. Lightly tighten your abdominal muscles.

Action

Keep your low back flat (do not increase the depth of your lumbar curve) and breathe in deeply while reaching overhead with the stick (*see* fig 9.4). Pause in the upper, fully stretched, position and then lower.

Tips

If the low back is allowed to move, the lumbar spine will hyperextend, taking some of the stretch away from the ribcage.

Focused inspiration – flat hand

Purpose

To expand the ribcage at the level of an injury.

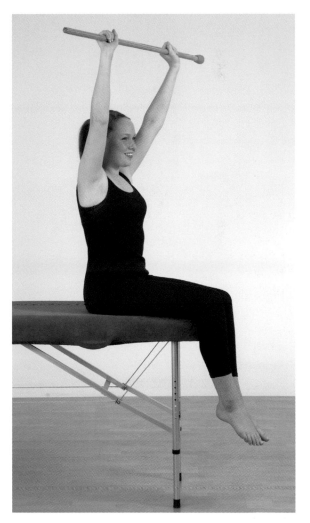

Figure 9.4 Deep breathing with arms raised

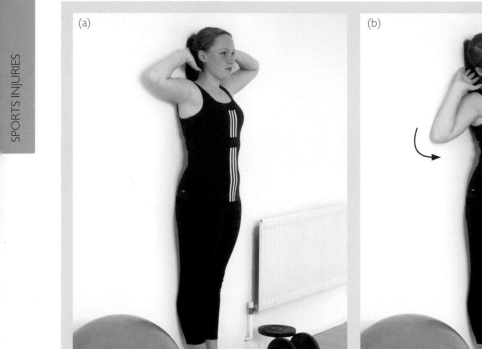

Figure 9.5 Standing side bend: (a) start position (b) side bend – point your top elbow towards the ceiling

Preparation
Sit on a gym bench or firm chair. Place the flat of your opposite hand over the area of your ribcage that was injured.

Action
Breathe in deeply and press your ribcage out against you hand. Hold the point of maximum inspiration for 5 seconds and then release. Breathe normally for 20–30 seconds and then repeat for 3–5 reps.

Tips
If your injury was to the back of your ribs, use a flat belt or thin towel wrapped around your chest at the level of injury. As you breathe in, press your ribs outwards against the belt.

Standing side bend
Purpose
To move the rib joints maximally using side bending to correct asymmetry.

Preparation

Begin standing with your back against a wall. Place your hands behind your head, or the backs of your hands on your forehead (*see* fig 9.5a, page 140).

Action

Breathe in and side bend, keeping your elbows back (aim to scrape the wall with your elbows). At the top of the movement, point your top elbow to the ceiling (*see* fig 9.5b, page 140).

Tips

The action is to open your ribcage rather than bend to your side. Your upper body should pivot around your breastbone (sternum). Done correctly, your breastbone should stay central rather than moving to one side.

Trunk rotation (with overpressure on elbows)

Purpose

To move the rib joints maximally using rotation to correct asymmetry.

Preparation

Begin sitting upright on a firm chair or gym bench. Loosely fold your arms and cup your hands under your elbows.

Action

Turn your upper body to the right (*see* fig 9.6). At the end of the movement range, pull a little further using your right hand to draw your left elbow around with your trunk. Pause at the end of the movement to emphasise the stretch and then release. Repeat the action to the left. Perform 3–5 reps to each side.

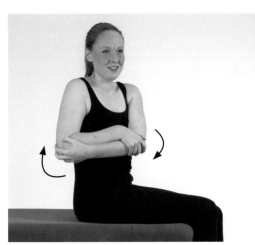

Figure 9.6 Trunk rotation (with overpressure on elbows)

Tips

Make sure that you sit up straight as this will enable your spine to move unhindered. If you sit round shouldered, your thoracic spine will bend forwards (flex), restricting the amount of rotation movement available to you.

TRAPPED NERVE

The nerves from your neck travel into the shoulder and down your arm into your fingers. Pain, tingling, weakness or just 'funny feelings' in your arm could therefore be the result of a neck injury. Nerves can be trapped if the spinal discs are injured, or placed under pressure when joints swell. In addition tight muscles and trigger points (painful nodules within a muscle) can also cause pain to travel (refer) some distance away from the original injury site. As we have seen in chapter 8, nerves should also move (slide) freely as you bend and stretch. After injury this natural movement can be restricted giving neural (nerve) tension.

Keypoint

Pain in your arm or hand may be coming from your neck.

Physiotherapists often use a special neural assessment called the *upper limb tension test* (ULTT), which combines neck rotation away from the arm with shoulder depression (shoulder blade pushed down), arm straightening, and wrist and hand movement. Depending on which movements cause pain or tingling, the particular nerve affected can be targeted. In addition, the ULTT can be converted to a neural stretch to lengthen the nerve and restore its normal sliding function.

When nerves are trapped you will tend to try to protect the area and alter your head-neck posture (*see* fig 9.7). Long after the pain has gone, your posture may still be altered, leaving you open to further problems. In addition, postural pain is a common syndrome in itself. Neck pain and headaches often have a component of poor posture, so postural correction has an important part to play in both prevention and treatment in this body area.

HEAD AND NECK POSTURE

The most common postural change in the neck is called a *head held forwards* (HHF) posture or *poking chin* (*see* fig 9.7, page 143). Normally there is a gentle curve in your neck which matches that in your low back. In the case of the low back (*see* chapter 8) this is called the *lumbar lordosis*, and in the neck it is the *cervical lordosis*. The cervical lordosis should be quite shallow, with the curve

going through the whole of the neck and the head held on the vertical posture line. Normally, if you imagine a long earring hanging down, the line should pass behind your collar bone. In the HHF posture this line passes in front of the collar bone through the upper chest. The head is too far forwards, and to get into this position the neck curve has not just increased, but it has become uneven. The chin pokes forwards so that the curve close to the top of the neck (upper cervical region) bends back markedly and the lower neck area (lower cervical region) bends further forwards than normal. The result is a dramatic increase in pressure to the upper cervical region, with the tissues becoming tight and painful. Stretching out this tight area and reversing the chin poke posture is a primary aim of treatment.

Keypoint

The most common postural change in the neck is a *poking chin*, also called *head held forwards* (HHF).

NECK AND SHOULDER MASSAGE

Massage to this area must be given with the head supported, otherwise the neck muscles will remain tense. Head support can be achieved with your partner either lying on their front with a folded towel beneath their forehead, or sitting and leaning forwards onto a high table.

Begin using stroking actions from the mid (thoracic) spine to the base of the skull and then down and out to the tips of the shoulders. This follows the location of the large trapezius muscle, which is often a source of pain in its upper areas

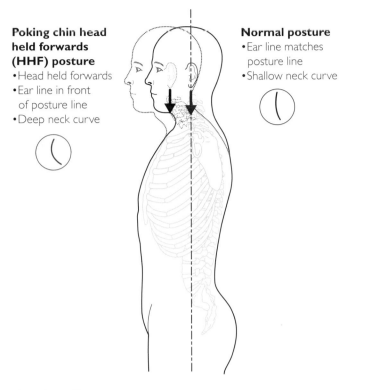

**Poking chin head
held forwards
(HHF) posture**
• Head held forwards
• Ear line in front
  of posture line
• Deep neck curve

Normal posture
• Ear line matches
  posture line
• Shallow neck curve

Figure 9.7 Altered head-neck position

(*see* fig 9.8a, page 144). Local massage may be given along the sides of the upper spine and neck using the fingertips. As you approach the top of the neck and the area narrows, you may find it easier to use the thumb and fingers (*see* fig 9.8b, page 144).

The neck muscles attach right up onto the base of the skull. This area often holds tension from a HHF posture, and is more easily accessed by standing at the head of your partner. Use your fingertips to grip lightly into the tissues on the base of the skull, drawing them towards you (*see* fig 9.8c, page 144). Strangely, pulling the hair gently will also help to reduce tension in the tissues

by releasing the skull fascia (the tissue between the skin and skull bone).

EXERCISES

Chin tuck with overpressure
Purpose
To relieve pain and correct a poking chin posture.

Preparation
Begin sitting upright in a firm-backed chair. Your upper back should touch the chair back (*see* fig 9.9a, overleaf).

SPORTS INJURIES

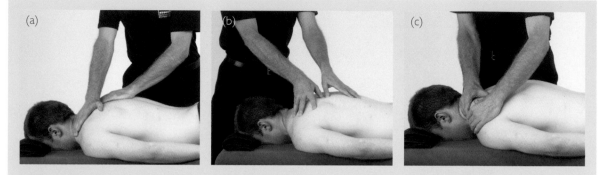

Figure 9.8 Neck and shoulder massage techniques: (a) stroking (b) local pressure (c) picking up

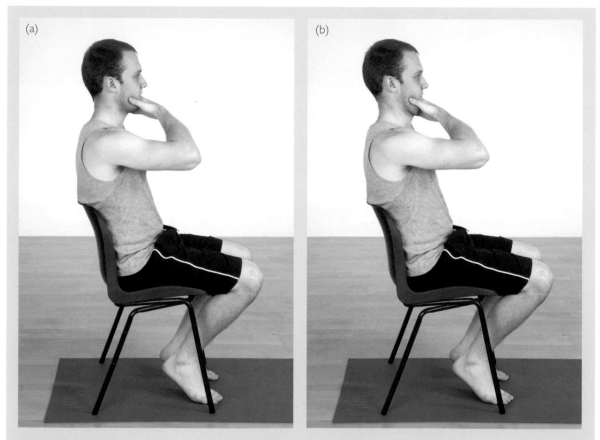

Figure 9.9 Chin tuck with overpressure: (a) start position (b) press the chin further inwards

Action

Keep looking forwards and draw your chin inwards, trying to give yourself a double chin. When you get as far as you can, gently press your chin further inwards using your fingers on your chin (*see* fig 9.9b, page 144). Pause in the inward position and then relax, allowing your chin to return to its original forward position. Repeat the action rhythmically for 10 reps.

Tips

If you have pain travelling into your shoulder or arm, this exercise should centralise your pain. This means that your pain reduces back into the neck where it has come from. For example, during the first few reps your pain may travel to your elbow; for the next reps, only to your shoulder; and finally, only into your neck. This is an indication that pressure on your nerve from your neck may be reducing.

Assisted neck rotation
Purpose

To increase the neck twisting (rotation) movement and restore symmetry.

Preparation

Begin sitting upright in a firm-backed chair. Your upper back should touch the chair back.

Action

Turn your head to the right. When you get as far as you can gently press on your jaw with your left hand to try to increase the movement by 0.5–1.0 cm. Hold the end position for a count of three and then return to the starting position. Turn to the left, this time pressing on your jaw with your right hand. Perform 5 reps each side.

Tips

Make sure that you sit upright   don't allow your chin to poke forwards.

Skull rock
Purpose

To mobilise the upper cervical spine using a nodding (flexion) action.

Preparation

Begin sitting upright in a firm-backed chair. Your upper back should touch the chair back (*see* fig 9.10a, page 146).

Action

Nod your head as though placing your chin into the notch at the top of your breastbone (jugular notch) (*see* fig 9.10b, page 146). The action should be to look down at your breastbone, not your knees. Your chin should stay in throughout the movement. Perform 5 reps and then rest.

Tips

It sometimes helps to imagine that you have a pin travelling through both ears, and that the pin acts as a pivot around which movement occurs.

WHIPLASH

Whiplash is usually associated with a car accident, but can actually occur in sport as well. It occurs when your body motion is suddenly stopped and your head continues to move. The action can cause considerable force on your neck, with damage to the delicate neck tissues. In medicine, whiplash has five grades (*see* table 9.1) from 0, where a whiplash has occurred but you have no symptoms at all, to 5, where there is a broken neck bone (fracture) or injury to the spinal cord itself

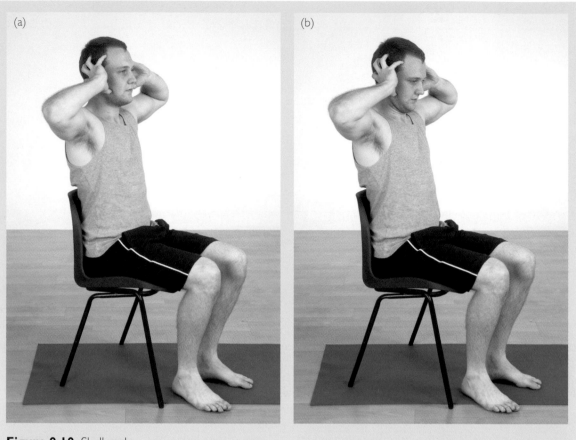

Figure 9.10 Skull rock

seen on an X-ray or scan. Often, following a whiplash, pain can occur some time after the accident, so it is important to see a physiotherapist to have your neck assessed. You may develop slight numbness in your fingers, for example, and not realise this for some time. The earlier this is caught, the easier it is to treat.

CONCUSSION

Concussion must be taken seriously because it is an injury affecting the brain. It occurs when the brain is rapidly shaken, for example during a collision between two players or when falling from a bicycle or horse. You may not notice that you have been unconscious, but will often feel dazed or simply 'not feel right'. Importantly, there is no damage to the brain tissues, and the injury is said to be a functional disturbance (things just not working correctly) rather than a structural disorder (tissue damage). Two types of concussion are generally seen: *simple* and *complex*. Simple concussion will generally get better in 7–10 days with rest, but complex concussion is said to be present when your symptoms persist or recur after 10 days.

Table 9.1	Grades of whiplash neck injuries
Grade	**Symptoms**
0	You suffered an injury but now have no neck pain, stiffness or other signs at all.
1	You feel neck pain occasionally but there is nothing apparent when examined (*no physical signs*).
2	You feel pain, and your physio finds pain when touching your neck (*point tenderness*) and stiffness when trying to turn it (*decreased range of motion*).
3	You have neck pain and signs that a nerve is trapped (*altered tendon response* or *sensory deficit*).
4	There is a change seen on X-ray or scan.

Table 9.2	Simplified Sports Concussion Assessment Tool (SCAT)	
Symptoms	*Does the player have any of the following:*	
	Loss of consciousness	Sensitivity to light or noise
	Convulsions	Just does not 'feel him/herself'
	Loss of memory	Difficulty concentrating or remembering
	Feelings of pressure in the head	Feels slow or has low energy level
	Neck pain	Feels drowsy or confused
	Feels sick or has thrown up	Feels anxious or irritable
	Dizziness	Feels emotional or sad
	Altered vision	
Memory	*Can the player answer all of the following:*	
	Where are we today?	
	Which half of the game is it?	
	Which team scored last – us or them?	
	Which team did we play last time?	
	Did our team win the last game?	
Balance	Ask the player to stand with one foot in front of the other (heel touching toe). Have them put their hands on their hips and close their eyes. Ask them to hold the position for 20 seconds. Concussion may be present if they make more than 5 errors (open eyes, lose balance, put arms out).	

Keypoint

Where a concussion is suspected: (i) accompany the player to hospital; (ii) do not leave them alone; and (iii) do not allow them to drive.

Because the brain is affected, any player colliding with another should be removed from the field and assessed using a SCAT chart, the acronym standing for *Sport Concussion Assessment Tool*.

Table 9.2 shows a simplified version of the SCAT chart and the full chart is available as a free download at http://www.sarugby.co.za/boksmart/pdf/PocketSCAT2%20final.pdf.

If a concussion is suspected the player should be taken to hospital and *never* left alone or allowed to drive.

Terms you should know:

Concussion – functional disturbance of the brain.

Referred pain – pain travelling from one body part to another.

SCAT – sport concussion assessment tool

Sublux – to partially dislocate, where one bone of a joint moves off the other.

Upper limb tension test (ULTT) – test of nerve tightness or involvement in the arm and shoulder.

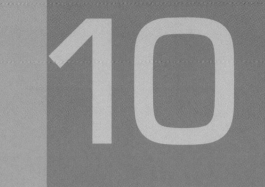

SHOULDER

The shoulder region actually consists of four joints (*see* fig 10.1). The upper arm bone (humerus) joins the shoulder blade (scapula) through the main ball and socket joint. The socket is actually called the *glenoid* and so the joint's official name is the *gleno-humeral joint*. The shoulder blade lies flat on the ribcage, forming the *scapulo-thoracic joint*, and, as we will see later, movements of these two are intimately linked. When the movement breaks down (becomes dysfunctional), pain often results.

The arm is held away from the body by the collar bone (clavicle), which acts as a strut. At either end it has a joint. On the outside it makes a joint with a beak of bone jutting forwards from the top of the shoulder blade called the *acromion process*. The joint here is called the *acromioclavicular (A/C) joint*, which is injured in the classic 'sprung shoulder' in rugby. Finally, on the inside of the clavicle, we have the *sternoclavicular (S/C) joint*, which can be injured through dipping exercises in the gym.

SHOULDER IMPINGEMENT

Shoulder impingement is a common condition that both gives pain directly, and often underlies other shoulder problems such as frozen shoulder, tendinopathy and instability. Essentially,

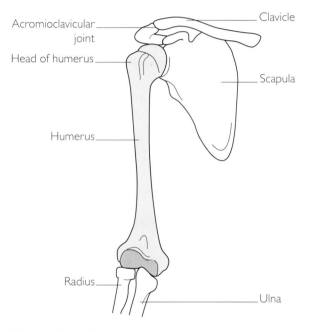

Figure 10.1 The shoulder joints

impingement means trapping, and a body structure becomes trapped between the upper arm bone and the structures which form the roof of the shoulder joint (coracoacromial arch). The two structures which are most commonly trapped are the tendon of the supraspinatus muscle and the long tendon of the biceps muscle. To

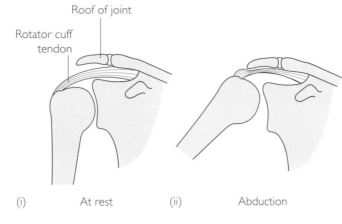

Roof of joint

Rotator cuff tendon

(i)   At rest   (ii)   Abduction

Figure 10.2 Shoulder impingement

understand this condition we first need to look at what happens when you raise your arm above your head – the so-called *abduction cycle*.

ABDUCTION CYCLE

One of the main problems the shoulder has is that the ball is too big for the socket. Because of this we have two sets of muscles. The first set, called the *rotator cuff* (*see* fig 10.2), lie close to the joint and work to hold the centre of the ball in the socket – they are the shoulder *stabilisers*. These continually adjust the position of the ball within the socket as we reach forwards or overhead, and, importantly, act to hold the two parts of the joint together. The second set of muscles are the shoulder movement muscles – the *mobilisers* – which you see when you look in the mirror. These are the muscle forming the cap of the shoulder (deltoid), the chest muscle (pectoral) and the shoulder span muscle (trapezius). For the shoulder to function correctly, the muscles must be *balanced* in terms of strength and stretch, and *coordinated* so that the right muscle works at the right time.

> **Keypoint**
> Health of the shoulder relies on balance and coordination between all the shoulder muscles. When this breaks down, pain is often the result.

As you lift your arm the shoulder cap muscle (deltoid) pulls the upper arm bone upwards, closer to the roof of the joint, actually making impingement more likely. To balance this, the rotator cuff muscles draw the ball of the joint downwards and inwards, reducing the chance of impingement and stabilising the joint (*see* fig 10.3, page 151). Providing you have a balance between the strength of your rotator cuff muscles and the other shoulder muscles, and providing the rotator cuff muscles work at the start of the movement and continue to work, your shoulder will function correctly and you will be pain free. However, commonly we have tightness at the front of the shoulder through our day-to-day posture from, for example, working on computers. As well as working to position the shoulder bones, the rotator cuff muscles now have to pull against this postural tightness and so fail to do their job correctly. Poor shoulder posture is therefore an important consideration in shoulder conditions.

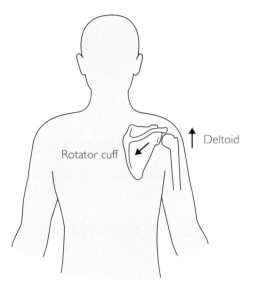

Rotator cuff

Deltoid

Figure 10.3 The balance of pull between deltoid and rotator cuff muscles during impingement

TRIGGER POINT RELEASE

Impingement often results in trigger points forming in the rotator cuff muscles, which remain for sometime after the impingement has cleared. The trigger points can occur quite quickly through something fairly innocent. You may sleep awkwardly, pressing the ball of the joint onto the cuff tendon, or go for an overhead shot in badminton and happen to tweak the tendon. Either of these can cause a small amount of swelling and pain which switches off the muscle (inhibition) temporarily to protect it. During this

time you are open to further injury because the abduction cycle will change.

To release the trigger point you can use a massage technique on your partner called *ischaemic release*. Here, you press your fingers deeply into the painful area and hold the pressure for 30–60 seconds. This presses fluids out of the tissues, and as you release your fingers fresh fluids flood back in, clearing the area of chemical waste products formed at the trigger point. To locate the trigger point, find the point of bone at the top of the shoulder blade (superior angle) and trace your finger inwards and downwards to find a ridge of bone called the *scapular spine*. Above this, you will find the *supraspinatus* muscle and below, the *infraspinatus*.

MASSAGE

General massage may be used to the back of the shoulder, to target the muscles around the shoulder blade, and to the front of the shoulder, to work on the rotator cuff attachments (*see* also fig 9.8, page 144). With your partner lying on their front, and their arms by their sides, locate the shoulder blade. It forms a triangle, with a vertical edge lying three finger-widths from the spine (*see* fig 10.4, overleaf). Along this inner edge are the *rhomboid* muscles which draw the shoulder blades together. At the top inner corner of the triangle (superior angle), the *levator* muscle attaches going to the base of the neck, and a trigger point is often found just off the bone. Cutting the scapula roughly in half in a diagonal is the scapula spine with the *supraspinatus* above it and the *infraspinatus* below. The thick muscle spanning the shoulder is the *trapezius* (middle fibres), which often has a trigger point midway between the spine and the point of the shoulder.

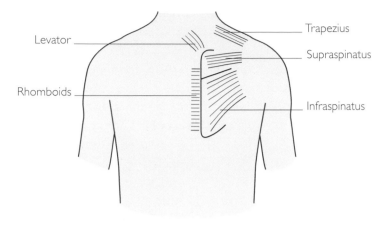

Figure 10.4 Muscle around the shoulder blade

After giving general stroking massage to aid relaxation, focus on the painful trigger points within these muscles using your fingertips or a massage tool. Following the massage, encourage your partner to move their shoulder blade up and down (shrugging) and inwards and outwards (bracing) to tense and relax the muscles.

Where impingement has occurred, the rotator cuff tendon will most commonly have been trapped at the front of the shoulder beneath the roof of the joint. This area can be targeted with deep transverse friction massage (DTF). To access the tendon your partner should be sitting at the front of a chair. Get them to place their hand behind their back on the painful side. The supraspinatus muscle rotates the shoulder outwards (lateral rotation) and placing the hand behind the back produces inward rotation (medial rotation) of the joint. This action therefore stretches the tendon, and reaching the arm backwards presses the ball of the joint forwards, drawing the tendon out from beneath the roof of the joint. Massage the tendon at the painful spot normally located just below the ball of the joint.

CORRECTION OF MOVEMENT DYSFUNCTION

One of the first things to do is to optimise the way the shoulder is working during the abduction cycle as you move your arm out sideways. If this hurts when you get close to the horizontal position, try to guide the joint to work properly. As mentioned earlier, the rotator cuff muscles should draw the ball of the socket down and back slightly to offset the action of the larger deltoid muscle, which as well as lifting the arm also pulls the ball of the joint upwards. If the rotator cuff has not worked properly for some time it will need to be re-educated. This is because the way that your shoulder now moves has become a habit even though the original injury may be long gone. This is a little like having a limp. If you get a stone in your shoe, you limp to avoid pressing the stone painfully into the sole of your foot. Over time this becomes a habit and you still limp even though the stone has been taken out. Similarly, movement dysfunction during impingement can be thought of as a 'limp' in your shoulder.

To correct this dysfunction you need to do the work of the rotator cuff muscles and draw your partner's shoulder back as they lift their arm. Get them to lift their arm unaided to begin with and register what this feels like. Then ask them to lift again as you guide the joint. If their pain reduces, the exercise will work.

Taping

Tape may be used to draw the ball of the joint backwards and remind your partner of the action practised during the movement dysfunction correction.

- Begin by placing a mesh underwrap over the shoulder from the front of the joint diagonally over the top of the shoulder to the lower inner point of the shoulder blade (inferior angle of the scapula).

- Place one or two pieces of non-elastic tape over the underwrap, beginning on the front of the shoulder and pulling the tape tight (up and back) as you attach it to the shoulder blade region (see fig 10.5).

EXERCISES

Guided arm lift
Purpose
To reduce pain from impingement and re-educate movement.

Preparation
Begin standing behind your partner. For right-sided pain, cup your right hand over their right shoulder and place your left hand over their shoulder blade.

Action
Ask them to raise their arm out to the side. As they do so, draw their shoulder backwards slightly by pulling on your right hand. At the same time, press the flat of your left hand gently against their shoulder blade to push it onto their ribcage. Perform 3–5 reps and then relax.

Tips
Your hands should follow their shoulder as it moves. As their pain reduces, gradually pull less with your hands so their muscles do more. Stop if there is any pain. Ease the pressure off until eventually you monitor scapular position with one finger and simply rest your other hand on top of their shoulder as a guide (see fig 10.6, overleaf). Stop if there is any pain.

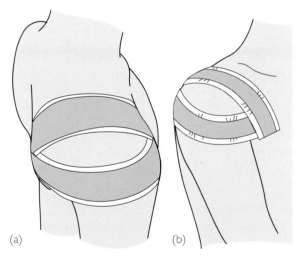

(a) (b)

Figure 10.5 Shoulder taping: (a) top view – shoulder taping begins over the front (anterior) aspect of the joint (b) front view – two pieces of tape are used finishing over the point of the shoulder blade (inferior angle of scapula)

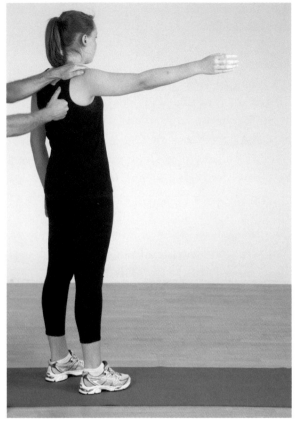

Figure 10.6 Guided arm lift

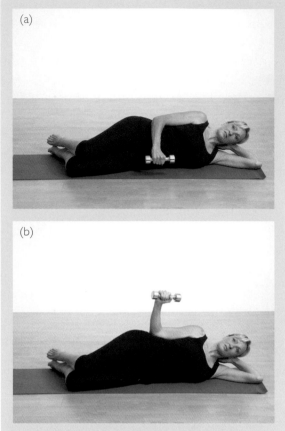

Figure 10.7 Lateral rotation with dumbbell:
(a) start position (b) mid position

Lateral rotation with dumbbell

Purpose
To strengthen the supraspinatus muscle.

Preparation
To exercise your right arm, lie on your left side. Hold a light (2 kg) dumbbell in your right hand and tuck your right elbow into your side (*see* fig 10.7a).

Action
Keeping your upper arm (humerus bone) in contact with your ribs, twist your arm (lateral rotation) to move your forearm towards the vertical position (*see* fig 10.7b). Lift as high as you can, holding the top position for 2–3 seconds and then lower slowly. Perform 5–8 reps and then rest.

Tips
If you allow your elbow to lift away from your ribcage, the exercise is less effective as work is taken away from the supraspinatus muscle.

Abduction with lateral rotation using a band

Purpose

To work the shoulder stabilising muscles (rotator cuff) and movement muscles (deltoid especially) at the same time.

Preparation

Begin holding a band with its lower end attached to the bottom of a door or low point.

Action

Raise your arm out sideways (abduction) and turn your arm outwards so your thumb faces the ceiling (lateral rotation) (*see* fig 10.8). Stop when you reach the horizontal position and then lower. Perform 8–10 reps and then rest.

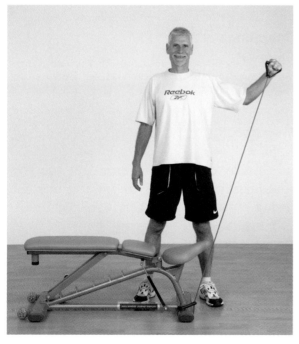

Figure 10.8 Abduction with lateral rotation using a band

Tips

Initially, lift your arm only to the horizontal position. As you improve, increase the movement range until you can lift overhead. You may find it easier and less painful to lift the arm forwards (20 degrees to the body plane) and upwards.

INSTABILITY

Shoulder instability means that your arm ball is too loose in its socket. The instability can be from a combination of three factors: *structure*, *injury* and *muscle action* (movement dysfunction) (*see* fig 10.9, page 156).

Structural factors include a shallow shoulder socket and a loose joint capsule. Injury may tear the rotator cuff muscles (supporting the joint), the ligaments or the capsule. As we have seen the rotator cuff muscles control the ball within its socket during movement, so if they do not work correctly instability may result.

Keypoint

Shoulder instability may come from injury, shoulder structure, or movement dysfunction.

All three of these factors work together, and where one is poor the other two can take over. So, for example a shoulder taping or brace can assist the structure of the joint and is useful when you are recovering from an injury. Surgery can repair tears and correct bone defects, which again fall into the structural category. Where injuries have recovered, it is vital to get the muscles working again and improve shoulder stability.

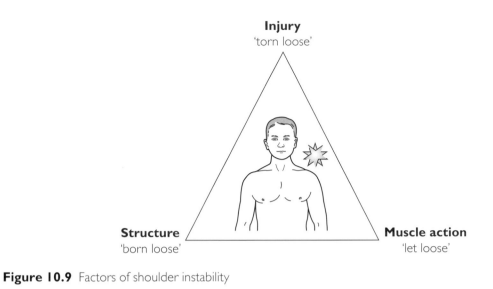

Injury
'torn loose'

Structure
'born loose'

Muscle action
'let loose'

Figure 10.9 Factors of shoulder instability

TAPING

Taping is used to draw the ball of the humerus up and back into its socket. Three pieces of tape are used over the large deltoid muscle, which caps the shoulder (*see* fig 10.10, page 157).

- Begin at the side of the shoulder and place a single piece of underwrap from the mid arm to the top of the shoulder.

- The second tape runs from the front of the shoulder and over the top to the shoulder blade.

- The third piece runs from the back of the shoulder inwards and over the top to the base of the neck.

- Non-elastic tape is placed on top and each piece is pulled upwards as though pulling the ball back into the socket.

EXERCISES

Scapular setting
Purpose
To strengthen the muscles holding the shoulder blade to the ribcage.

Preparation
Begin with your partner lying on their front. For left shoulder pain, stand on their right side. Cup your right hand beneath the front of their left shoulder. Your left hand should be placed flat over their right shoulder blade.

Action
Draw their shoulder blade towards you (shoulder ball off the bench), inwards to their spine and downwards to their waist (*see* fig 10.11, page 157). Perform this action twice and then get them to follow your movement drawing their shoulder blade in and down.

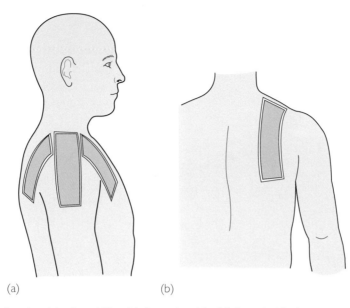

Figure 10.10 Taping for shoulder instability: (a) from the side (b) from behind

Tips

As your partner improves, reduce the pull from your hands. Begin quite forcefully to stretch the tight front shoulder structures and gradually release the tension to change from stretching to guiding the movement.

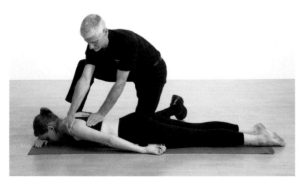

Figure 10.11 Scapular setting

Hand walking – kneeling

Purpose

To enhance shoulder stability and control.

Preparation

Begin kneeling on all fours on a gym mat.

Action

Taking most of your weight on your knees, walk your hands forwards and backwards one at a time, moving 20–30 cm with each hand step. As you gain confidence move your weight forwards over your hands and away from your knees (*see* fig 10.12, page 158).

Tips

The exercise can be made harder by hand stepping on and off a shallow step or block.

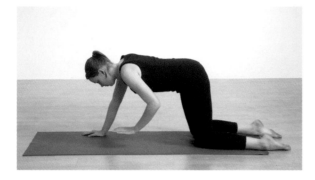

Figure 10.12 Hand walking – kneeling

Press-up position on a balance board
Purpose
To build shoulder stability and control.

Preparation
Begin in the press-up position with hands 0.5 m apart, and a balance board (wobble board) between your hands (*see* fig 10.13).

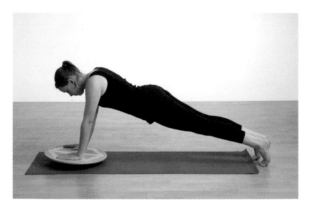

Figure 10.13 Press-up position on a balance board

Action
Place one hand in the centre of the balance board and lean your weight onto this hand. Hold for 8–10 seconds, trying to keep the rim of the board off the ground. Repeat with the other hand. Rest for 1 minute and then first place your right hand and then your left hand either side of the centre of the board. Hold for 8–10 seconds, again trying to keep the rim of the board off the ground.

Tips
If you find this exercise too hard on your wrists, perform it from kneeling on all fours (4-point kneeling) rather than the press-up position (officially called prone falling). Lean forwards from kneeling to press your bodyweight onto your hands.

Cuban press with dumbbells
Purpose
To work the rotator cuff and shoulder abductor muscles intensely.

Preparation
Begin standing holding a light (2 kg) dumbbell in each hand. Bend your elbows and raise them to shoulder level so your upper arms are horizontal and your forearms are near vertical, pointing downwards, knuckles facing forwards (see fig 10.14a, page 159).

Action
First, keeping your upper arms horizontal, swivel your forearms through 180 degrees (shoulder lateral rotation) so your forearms point vertically upwards (knuckles face backwards) (*see* fig 10.14b, page 159). Next, press the dumbbells overhead, aiming to touch your upper arms to your ears (*see* fig 10.14c, page 159). Lower until your upper arms are horizontal again, with knuckles facing backwards. Swivel your forearms down so your knuckles face forwards to complete one rep. Perform 5 reps and then rest.

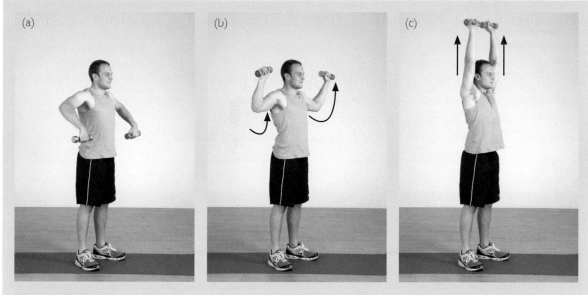

Figure 10.14 Cuban press with dumbbells: (a) start position (b) mid position (c) finish position

Tips

This is a complex action. If you find the coordination difficult, split the movement into two. Perform 5 reps of the first action and then rest. Next, perform 5 reps of the second action, beginning with your knuckles facing back. Rest once more and then perform 5 reps of the complete action.

FROZEN SHOULDER

Frozen shoulder (adhesive capsulitis) is a stiffening of the shoulder joint. The condition can occur spontaneously or follow on from an untreated instability or rotator cuff tendinopathy. The shoulder is a very flexible joint, and, like any other fluid-filled (synovial) joint, it is surrounded by a bag called the *capsule* and this in turn is strengthened by reinforcing ligaments. The bottom of the capsule in the shoulder is folded a little like a bellows with the folds opening up to allow a high degree of movement without the capsule hanging loose. With a frozen shoulder, the capsule thickens and tightens with the folds sticking together. Ligaments at the front of the joint tighten and the space between two of the rotator cuff tendons, supraspinatus and subscapularis, at the front of the joint (rotator interval) is lost. The condition is accompanied by muscle spasm and trigger point formation, and reducing these often results in some of the movement returning.

Where trigger points are present, specific massage and local stretching exercises can be useful. In chronic cases where no movement has been available for months or even years, a capsular release operation may be required to cut through strands of scarring which form around the joint. After surgery, exercise is again required.

A frozen shoulder gives both pain and stiffness and is normally described in three stages, with treatment tailored to each phase. In stage (i), pain is the dominant feature, with movement limited by mainly muscle spasm. The joint capsule at this stage is normal but the joint may be slightly inflamed. The main aim at this stage is to ease pain and you can used gentle pendular swinging exercise to help (*see* opposite). If the frozen shoulder continues, after about 3–6 months it can progress to stage (ii), where stiffness increases. The joint capsule changes from being elastic and healthy to being dull and leathery, with scarring beginning to form between the joint structures. Stretching exercise can be used now, but it should be gentle – don't press as far as you can (end range). If too much stretching is practised the joint will flare up and pain will increase, so *encourage* movement rather than force it. In stage (iii), pain begins to reduce, although this can take up to 9 months. As pain recedes, stretching can increase and you can press the joint to full range actions.

Keypoint

In the early stages of a frozen shoulder (0–3 months), avoid painful actions as they can worsen the condition. Later (3–9 months), *mild pain* from stretching can be expected. Where *severe pain* occurs, the exercise is too intense.

EXERCISES

Let's look at some exercises you can use with a frozen shoulder. Remember, however, that you must not exercise through increasing pain. If a stretch hurts slightly and the pain reduces, that is fine because you are feeling the stretching intensity. If pain increases, the joint is reacting and so you should stop. Rest for a while and then try again.

Pendular swinging
Purpose
To reduce pain in the shoulder.

Preparation
Begin leaning over, with your unaffected arm straight on a table top and your affected arm hanging free. To further draw the shoulder ball away from its socket, add the use of a weight around your wrist (*see* fig 10.15, page 161).

Action
Gently begin to circle your painful arm, keeping it straight (*see* fig 10.15, page 161). Your hand should move in a circle approximately 20 cm in diameter. Sway your body to create power for the movement, trying to relax your shoulder muscles as much as possible. Allow the weight of your arm to draw the ball of the joint away from the socket slightly. Continue for 1–2 minutes and practise 3–4 times each day.

Tips
The more you can relax your shoulder muscles and use your body sway to perform the movement the better.

Shoulder traction – kneeling
Purpose
To traction (pull) the shoulder joint.

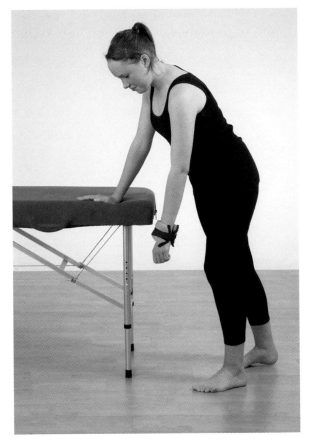

Figure 10.15 Pendular swinging

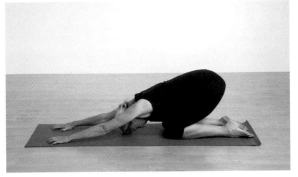

Figure 10.16 Shoulder traction – kneeling

Tips

This action both tractions your shoulder joint and presses your arm overhead. The overhead action is emphasised by pressing your chest down to the floor. Traction is emphasised by walking your knees further back and sitting towards your heels.

Hands behind back, hands behind head

Purpose

To increase rotation (twisting) range on the shoulder joint.

Preparation

Begin standing with your feet shoulder width apart.

Action

Place your hands behind your back (shoulder medial rotation) and draw your elbows back (*see* fig 10.17a, page 161). Hold the position for 3–5 seconds and then rest. Next, place your hands behind your head (shoulder lateral rotation) and draw your elbows back (*see* fig 10.17b, page 161). Again, hold the position for 3–5 seconds before resting. The whole cycle is 1 rep, and you should aim to perform 5 reps in total.

Preparation

Begin kneeling. Grip the floor tightly with your fingertips.

Action

Sit back towards your heels keeping your arms straight (*see* fig 10.16). Maintain the grip on the floor so your hands do not slide. Hold the end position for 10–20 seconds and then release. Perform 5 reps and then rest.

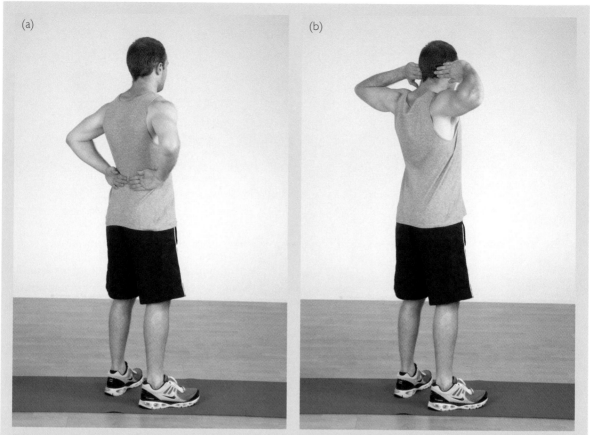

Figure 10.17 Hands behind back, hands behind head: (a) hands behind the back drawing elbows back (b) hands behind the head drawing elbows back

Tips

As you place your hands behind your back there is a tendency to round your shoulders – correct this by bracing your shoulders slightly.

Lateral rotation stretch

Purpose

To stretch the tissues at the front of your shoulder.

Preparation

Begin standing close to a wall or pillar. Hold your upper arm against your chest (elbow tucked in) and bend your elbow to 90 degrees (*see* fig 10.18a, page 163). Fix your hand against the wall.

Action

Turn your body away from your arm, pressing your arm into lateral rotation (*see* fig 10.18b, page 163). Hold the fully stretched position for 20–30 seconds and then release. Perform 3–5 reps.

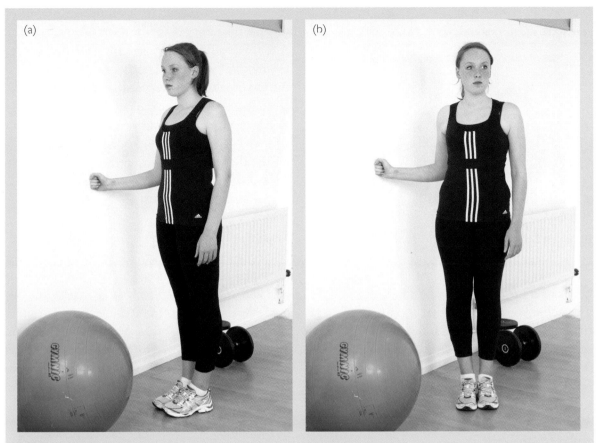

Figure 10.18 Lateral rotation stretch: (a) start position (b) turning the body to stretch the shoulder

Tips

If you allow your elbow to come away from your body the stretch is released.

Wall walking

Purpose

To increase shoulder movement range.

Preparation

Stand about 0.5 m away from a wall. Place your fingertips on the wall.

Action

Walk your fingers up the wall as high as you can and then walk them down again. Begin facing the wall (shoulder flexion) and then turn side on (shoulder abduction) (*see* fig 10.19, page 164).

Tips

Contracting your shoulder muscles when your arm is away from your body may be painful, so keep as much weight on your fingers as possible and relax your arm.

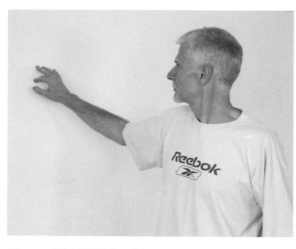

Figure 10.19 Wall walking

COLLAR BONE INJURY

The collar bone (clavicle) has a joint at each end: the A/C joint on the outside and the S/C joint on the inside. Both of these joints may be injured, but it is the A/C joint which is more commonly involved in a sprung shoulder injury. A more severe injury to the collar bone can result in a break (fracture).

> **Keypoint**
>
> A fall onto the shoulder or arm can disrupt the clavicle joints. More severe injury may cause a fracture.

SPRUNG SHOULDER

The A/C joint is fairly flat with weak ligaments. Any sudden force directly on it, or through the arm if you fall onto your hand, may disrupt the joint. If the force is quite small the joint may just swell and be painful, but if the force is larger –

such as when falling in horseriding, skiing or rugby – the joint may come apart (dislocate). The A/C dislocation is commonly called a *sprung shoulder* and you will notice a prominent lump on the top of your shoulder (a step deformity) where one bone rides up over the other. When you see a physiotherapist they will often gently pull your arm and if the A/C joint dislocates further it means that the ligaments surrounding the joint have snapped (ruptured) rather than just overstretched.

Taping

Initial treatment is to tape the joint to try to keep the bones closer together. This will help the tissue heal and reduce pain. The tape is applied in two parts: the first presses the A/C joint bones together and the second takes some of the weight of the arm.

As pulling on the arm increases the A/C dislocation in some cases, begin with your partner sitting with their elbow supported on a low table. This will shrug (elevate) the shoulder blade and will be more comfortable for them.

• Begin the taping using three pieces of underwrap, one from the front to the back of the chest below the nipple, and the second passing over the A/C joint, travelling between the ends of the first tape. The third piece of underwrap is placed around the upper arm.

• Place an adhesive felt pad over the A/C joint to compress it and stop the tape rubbing on the prominent bump.

• Next, apply non-elastic tape strips on top of the underwrap: the first piece around the chest, the second over the joint. Apply this second piece under some tension to press the A/C joint down.

- For the third tape, put one piece around the arm and then put two stirrups from the arm to the top of the shoulder. Pull this tape upwards to give support.

Leave the tape on for 3–4 days and then remove it. If the pain has gone then gentle exercise may begin, but if pain remains reapply the taping for 3–4 days once more.

FRACTURED COLLAR BONE

The collar bone may fracture with a very severe knock or fall. Treatment will be required at hospital, where the shoulders will be bandaged or the arm rested in a sling (collar and cuff) for about 3 weeks. In some cases a small operation is required to put a metal plate along the collar bone to support it.

When you have been discharged from hospital you will need to start gentle exercise.

EXERCISES

Begin using gentle pendular swinging as previously described to settle the pain and get the shoulder moving. Then progress the exercise for both general shoulder strength and mobility. Initially, begin with movements keeping the arm below the horizontal and eventually increase range.

Shoulder shrug
Purpose
To mobilise the shoulder blade and collar bone.

Preparation
Begin standing holding two dumbbells (*see* fig 10.20a, overleaf).

Action
Keep your arms straight and shrug your shoulders up towards your ears (shoulder elevation) (*see* fig 10.20b, overleaf). Relax and allow your shoulder to move down again (shoulder depression). Perform 10 reps.

Tips
Make sure you lift both shoulders equally, as your injured shoulder may be stiffer. Also, ensure that your shoulder lowers completely by relaxing the shoulder span muscles (trapezius).

Chair arm dip
Purpose
To strengthen the shoulder blade stabilising muscles.

Preparation
Begin sitting on a firm chair with arms. The chair should not swivel and the arms should be rigid and non-adjustable. Sit upright away from the chair back and place your hands on the chair arms.

Action
Push down with your hands to try to lift yourself up and out of the chair. Lift as high as you can, drawing your shoulders downwards (ears away from your shoulders). Hold the high position for 3–5 seconds and then release. Perform 5 reps.

Tips
It is important to press your shoulder blades down (shoulder depression), rather than just lifting yourself with your arm muscles (triceps).

Table slide
Purpose
To mobilise the shoulder and clavicle joints.

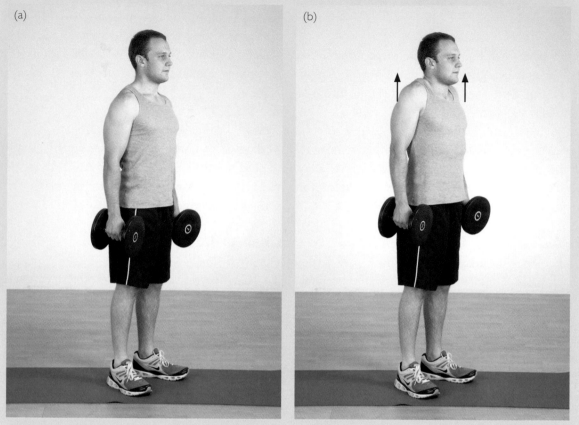

Figure 10.20 Shoulder shrug: (a) start position (b) mid position showing the lift of the shoulders

Preparation
Begin sitting facing a table with your hand resting on a cloth.

Action
Sliding your hand on the table surface, first reach forwards and backwards as far as you can (shoulder flexion). Next, stretch your arm forwards and, keeping it straight, sweep it from side to side (shoulder flexion-abduction). Finally, turn your body to sit side on to the table, and reach your arm out sideways (shoulder abduction).

Tips
Make sure you rest as much of your arm weight as possible on the table top to relax your shoulder muscles. As you perform the sweeping actions, gradually increase the amount of movement, working into the stiff range.

Assisted overhead reach
Purpose
To increase motion at the shoulder and improve strength.

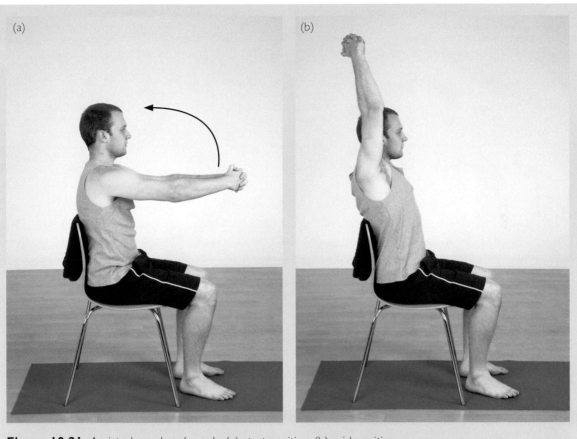

Figure 10.21 Assisted overhead reach: (a) start position (b) mid position

Preparation

Begin sitting on a firm-backed chair with your back tight up against the chair back. Interlace your fingers and straighten your arms (*see* fig 10.21a).

Action

Reach forwards and stretch your arms out (traction), encouraging the movement of your stiff arm with your unaffected arm. Keep the lengthened arm position and then gradually reach overhead as far as you can (*see* fig 10.21b). Hold the high position for 3–5 seconds and then lower, maintaining the feeling of arm lengthening.

Tips

The arm lengthening action should underlie all of the movements of this exercise to avoid the shoulder muscles 'bunching up' and going into protective spasm.

Pole press
Purpose

To maintain shoulder mobility and build functional strength.

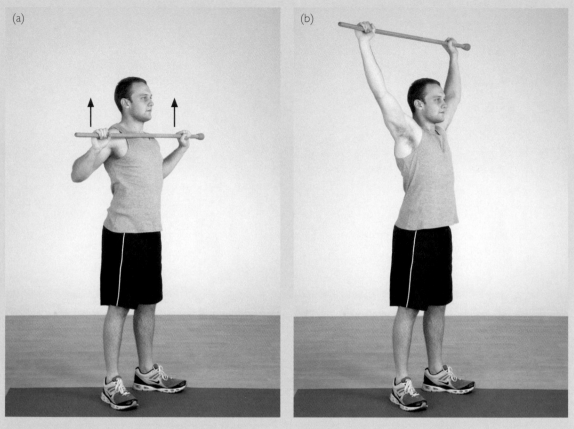

Figure 10.22 Pole press: (a) start position (b) mid position

Preparation

Begin standing with your feet shoulder width apart. Grip a pole (broom handle) in both hands, keeping your hands about 1.5 times shoulder width apart. Lift the pole onto the top of your chest with your palms facing upwards (*see* fig 10.22a).

Action

Press the pole straight upwards overhead, keeping your arms level with your ears (*see* fig 10.22b).

Lock your elbows out and then lower the bar back to your chest. Perform 10 reps.

Tips

As you press upwards, watch your posture: (i) your back should not overarch – tighten your abdominal muscles slightly; (ii) push equally with each arm; and (iii) the pole should be horizontal throughout the action – do not allow one side to dip. As you improve, exchange the pole for a barbell (no weights), and eventually a barbell with one 2 kg disc on each end.

Terms you should know:

Instability – excessive and uncontrolled movement of a body part.

Lateral rotation – twisting a limb away from the body (outwards).

Medial rotation – twisting a limb towards the body (inwards).

Movement muscle – muscle better at moving a body part.

Pendular swinging – swinging the arm using body momentum rather than shoulder muscle strength.

Scapular setting – gripping the shoulder blade tightly onto the ribcage.

Stabiliser muscle – muscle better at holding a body part tight and protecting it.

Synovial joint – joint which contains watery fluid.

ELBOW AND FOREARM

11

The elbow consists of three joints. The upper arm bone (humerus) forms joints with both the bone on the thumb side of the forearm (radius) and the bone on the little finger side of the forearm (ulna). The two forearm bones also form a joint to allow the radius bone to twist. Your elbow can therefore bend and straighten (flexion and extension) and swivel to face your palm down (pronation) or up (supination).

The forearm muscles are all long and lean and their tendons come together to attach to knobbles of bone on the inside and outside of the elbow. On the inside of the forearm this is called the *common flexor origin* (CFO) and on the outside, the *common extensor origin* (CEO). Both are involved in sports injuries to the elbow.

TENNIS ELBOW

Tennis elbow is a tendon condition (tendinopathy) affecting the CEO on the outside (back) of the elbow. Pain occurs when you grip and when you lift objects with your knuckles upwards (pronated position). The muscles commonly affected are the long (extensor carpi radialis longus) and short (extensor carpi radialis brevis) wrist extensor muscles. These muscles can be affected when they attach directly to the bone (an area called the *teno-osseous junction*), or a little further back within the muscle tendon itself (called the *musculotendinous junction*). If the bone is affected, you feel pain right on the knobble of bone at your elbow and sometimes slightly above the elbow joint. Where the tendon is affected, pain is within the cord-like tendon leading down from the elbow joint.

Pain is made worse if you lift your wrist up against a resistance and, where the shorter (brevis) muscle is affected, pain is even worse still when the third finger is lifted. Often you have been doing a repeated action such as racquet sports or a hammering action. Although you suddenly feel pain, this is frequently due to a background build-up over a number of weeks which comes to a head. The tissue around the elbow thickens and new blood vessels grow into it, in a type of uncontrolled or excessive healing (hyperplasia).

Keypoint

Hyperplasia (excessive healing) occurs when tissue cells multiply more rapidly than expected in response to injury or overuse.

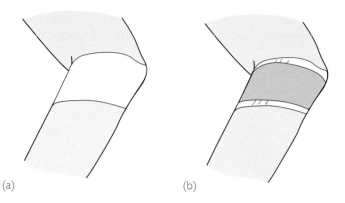

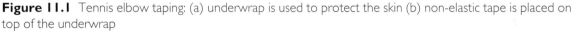

(a)   (b)

Figure 11.1 Tennis elbow taping: (a) underwrap is used to protect the skin (b) non-elastic tape is placed on top of the underwrap

Treatment aims to reduce pain by spreading the load on the elbow tissues with taping, changing the way you grip objects and subjecting the tissues to controlled loading to reset the healing process.

Occasionally, pain that appears to be tennis elbow can actually be coming from your neck. In this case there is little pain when the fingers or wrist are lifted against a resistance. Confirming that the neck is the problem rather than the elbow requires a physiotherapy examination to rule out nerve involvement.

TAPING AND GRIP CHANGE

Taping can be used to reduce pain from a tennis elbow by spreading the load across the forearm muscles.

- Apply underwrap just below your partner's elbow crease (*see* fig 11.1a).

- Place strips of non-elastic tape around two thirds of their elbow, pulling on the skin to unload the tissues (*see* fig 11.1b).

- As they grip, you should notice the muscles tighten beneath the taping and they should feel pain reduction.

A commercially available tennis elbow splint is also available, which is tightened and then closed using a hook-and-loop fastener. The advantage of a splint of this type is that it can be used when you are performing a gripping action and taken off between activities.

This taping may be modified to unload the elbow extensor muscles. For this, check first that unloading the tissues relieves pain. Have your partner grip a ball to determine their level of pain. When they have relaxed, dig your thumbs into the fleshy tissue bulk below their painful area (extensor muscle bellies), and press the tissues outwards (lateral glide). Have your partner grip the ball again. If pressing the tissues outwards reduces their pain, this second taping is likely to work; if not, the first taping method should be used.

- To unload the tissues, attach a strip of underwrap to the inner aspect of your partner's elbow and pull (glide) the tape outwards, stretching the extensor tissues sideways.

- Apply a piece of non-elastic tape over the underwrap and again pull the tissues outwards with greater force.

Using a wider (fatter) grip on an object also helps. When a narrow grip is used on a racquet the finger tendons are put on stretch. A wider grip takes some of the stretch off and so pain is reduced. Simply wrapping the handle of an object with foam rubber or using a padded cycling glove can give a surprising amount of pain relief. This is especially useful where the tennis elbow is aggravated by, for example, hammering or using spanners at work.

> **Keypoint**
> The size of an object being gripped is important in tennis elbow. A *wider* grip is generally more comfortable for this condition.

MASSAGE

Massage may be used along the extensor muscles to reduce pain. The muscles often develop painful trigger points, and targeting these can give substantial relief. Begin using circular finger pressure along the muscle from the bone on the outside of the elbow, along the forearm, to the wrist. As you find painful points, press these firmly and hold the pressure until the pain subsides (30–40 seconds). Repeat this process 3 or 4 times and finish with general stroking actions along the same area.

Specific work can be given using deep transverse friction (DTF) massage. For this the tendon should be placed on stretch by resting the forearm on a cushion and allowing the hand to drop over the end (wrist flexion) (*see* fig 11.2). The massage sweeps across the tendon, with your fingers and the skin moving as one. Begin quite gently, pressing more firmly as pain eases. Use the DTF for 3–5 minutes to stimulate the tissues adequately.

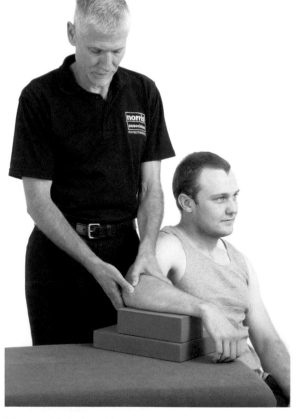

Figure 11.2 Specific work given using DTF massage

EXERCISES

Wrist extensor strengthening

Purpose

To strengthen the wrist extensor muscles on the back of the arm.

Preparation

Kneel behind a chair with your forearm supported by a folded towel on the back of the chair. Your hand should be over the end of the chair with your wrist bent (flexed) (*see* fig 11.3a). Wrap a cloth or thin towel around the handle of a 1–2 kg dumbbell, and grip the dumbbell in your affected hand.

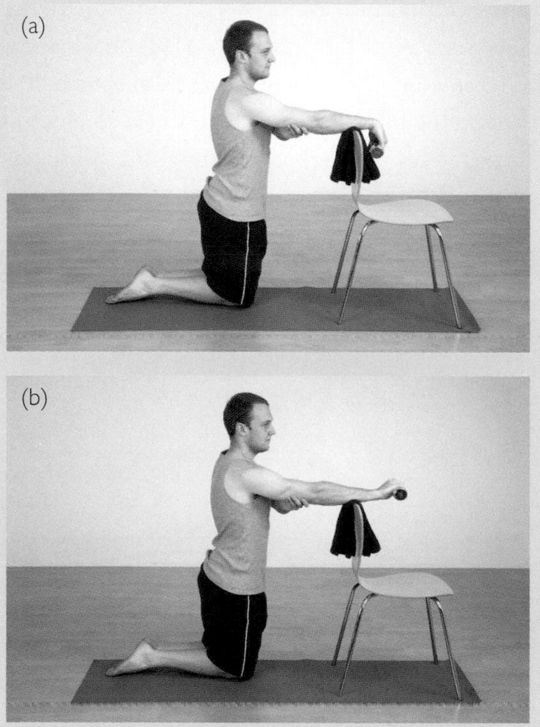

Figure 11.3 Wrist extensor strengthening: (a) start position – wrist bent (b) wrist extension

Action

Keeping your forearm still, lift your hand upwards as high as you can (wrist extension) (*see* fig 11.3b) and then lower back to the starting position. Perform 10 reps slowly, avoiding any rapid jarring movements.

Tips

To begin with, you may find the fully lifted position (end-range wrist extension) painful. Avoid this position to start with, but as pain eases gradually work further into this position.

Wrist extensor stretch

Purpose

To lengthen the wrist extensor muscles.

Preparation

Begin facing a wall with your affected arm held out straight, wrist bent (flexed). Place a folded towel between the back of your hand and the wall if you like. Lock your elbow and hold it locked with the cup of your unaffected hand.

Action

Lean forwards slightly to press the back of your hand against the wall, encouraging your wrist to bend (flex) maximally (*see* fig 11.4, overleaf). Hold the stretched position for 20–30 seconds and then slowly release.

Tips

Allowing your elbow to bend even slightly will release the stretch.

173

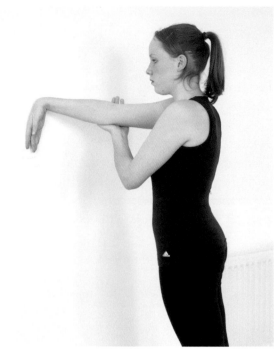

Figure 11.4 Wrist extensor stretch

Eccentric loading
Purpose
To stress the tissue affected by tennis elbow and encourage remodelling.

Preparation
Begin with your forearm resting on a block or cushions, with your hand over the end.

Action
Keeping your forearm on the block, lift your wrist back (extension). Pass a moderately heavy dumbbell (5–8 kg) from your unaffected hand to your affected one. Grip the dumbbell in the extended wrist position and lower the weight slowly. Release the dumbbell and lift it using

your unaffected hand once more. Perform 8–10 reps.

Tips
The idea of this exercise is that you use a dumbbell which would be too heavy for you to lift (concentric muscle work) but which you are able to lower under control (eccentric muscle work). This intense muscle work encourages the modified healing of the affected elbow tissues.

Mobilisation with movement (MWM)
Purpose
To reduce pain during gripping actions.

Preparation
Begin with your partner lying on their back on a bed or couch. The affected arm should be by their side, and they should grip a ball. Place your cupped hands above and below their elbow, with your lower hand (below the elbow) facing outwards and your upper hand (above the elbow) facing inwards (*see* fig 11.5).

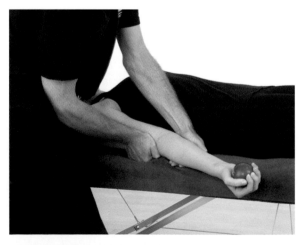

Figure 11.5 Mobilisation with movement

Action

Press your hands together, moving (gliding) your partner's forearm outwards and their upper arm inwards by 0.5–1.0 cm. At the same time they should grip the ball gently. Perform 8–10 reps, increasing the grip force on the ball as pain subsides.

Tips

Your hand pressure should be at 90 degrees to your partner's arm.

GOLFER'S ELBOW

Pain on the inside of the elbow is called *golfer's elbow* and affects the tendons on the underside of the forearm (especially pronator teres and flexor carpi radialis). Pain here must be differentiated from problems with the inner elbow ligament (medial collateral ligament). Golfer's elbow is painful when gripping and pulling the wrist upwards (flexion), while injury to the elbow inner ligament is more painful when the elbow is straight and levered open by pressing the forearm outwards while the upper arm stays still. This type of action occurs in throwing, for example, and can be reproduced when a physiotherapist assesses your elbow joint.

The nerve on the inside of the forearm (ulnar nerve) may also be affected. When this is the case your physiotherapist can use *Tinel's test*, where the nerve within a small groove on the inside of the elbow is gently tapped. If the nerve is affected it will be hypersensitive compared to the non-affected side and give a sensation of pins and needles (tingling) along the inner forearm and into your little finger.

MASSAGE

Massage is targeted at the inner aspect of the joint. Have your partner lie on their back with their arm straight. Press their wrist backwards (extension)

Keypoint

Golfer's elbow must be differentiated from pain from the inner elbow ligament, or pain from the ulnar nerve. A physiotherapist can use special tests to do this.

and massage from the inner elbow bone (medial epicondyle) down towards the little finger. Perform DTF massage using the forefinger supported by the ring finger. Move across the muscle tendon just below the prominent elbow bone. A tennis elbow splint may also be positioned to give relief from golfer's elbow by unloading the tissues.

EXERCISES

Resisted wrist flexion
Purpose

To strengthen the wrist flexor muscles.

Preparation

Begin kneeling in front of a gym bench with your affected forearm flat on the bench (palm upwards) and your hand over the bench side. Hold a light (2 kg) dumbbell in your hand (*see* fig 11.6a, overleaf).

Action

Bend your wrist backwards (extension) opening your fingers slightly to allow the dumbbell to roll down by 2–3 cm. Pull the hand back up, tightening your grip again, and bend the wrist forwards (flexion) (*see* fig 11.6b, overleaf). Perform 8–10 reps.

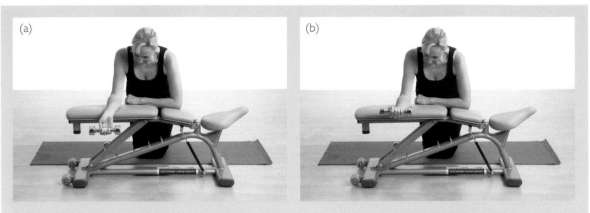

Figure 11.6 Resisted wrist flexion: (a) start position (b) mid position

Tips
Choose a dumbbell with a thick handle as it will be easier to grip.

Hammer pronation
Purpose
To strength the forearm pronator muscles.

Preparation
Begin with the elbow of your affected arm bent to 90 degrees (knuckles down) and tucked into the side of your body. Hold a hammer at the end of its handle, with the hammer head to the outside of your body (*see* fig 11.7).

Action
Twist your forearm downwards (pronation) so that your knuckles face upwards and the hammer head moves to the inside of your body. Pause and then move back to the starting position. Perform 8–10 reps.

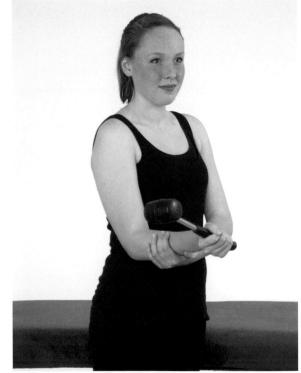

Figure 11.7 Hammer pronation

Tips

Begin with a small, light hammer. The leverage effect makes the exercise more difficult than it at first appears.

Forearm flexor stretch

Purpose

To stretch the forearm flexor muscles.

Preparation

Begin facing a wall with the elbow of your affected arm locked out, fingers pointing down. Hold the elbow straight with your opposite cupped hand (*see* fig 11.8).

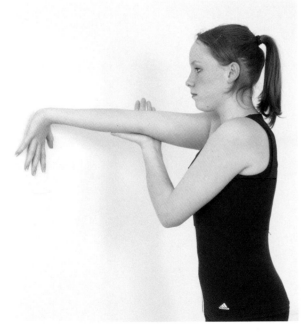

Figure 11.8 Forearm flexor stretch

Action

Lean forwards to press the heel of your hand onto the wall. Hold the stretched position for 10–20 seconds and then release. Perform 3–5 reps.

Tips

The stretch is greater when your hand is higher than your shoulder and less when your hand is towards your waist.

POSTERIOR ELBOW PAIN

Pain on the back of the elbow is common in throwing sports, pressing actions in the gym, and punching in martial arts where the elbow is locked out rapidly. At the back of the elbow, the inner elbow bone (ulna) joins onto the upper arm bone (humerus) as a U-shaped joint, with the point of the elbow (olecranon process) acting as the attachment for the powerful triceps muscle (*see* fig 11.9, overleaf). Separating the bone and triceps muscle is a fluid-filled sack or bursa (deep bursa). At the point of the elbow there is a larger bursa (superficial olecranon bursa). As you straighten your arm this bursa pulls on the skin, giving a circular ridge about 1.5 cm wide.

Repeated elbow-locking actions can cause inflammation to the triceps muscle attachment and the olecranon bursa, giving pain and swelling. As the joint snaps back, bone touches bone and the area can become very painful (posterior impingement) at the back and on the inner aspect of the back of the joint (postero-medial aspect). When examined by a physiotherapist your elbow will hurt as it is locked out and this pain gets even worse as your hand is pulled out sideways.

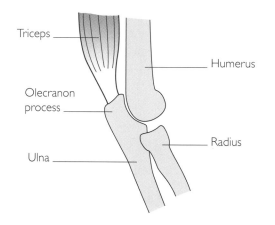

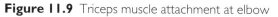

Figure 11.9 Triceps muscle attachment at elbow

Keypoint

Posterior impingement gives pain at the back of the elbow when the arm is snapped out straight.

It is essential that you rest from actions involving locking the elbow and protect your joint with a taping. Once pain has resolved, it is important to look at your sports actions to see if you can identify anything which may have given rise to the condition. Failure to change incorrect technique will often result in the injury coming back.

TAPING

An X-tape is used to prevent the elbow from locking out and take some stress away from the injured tissues (*see* fig 11.10).

• Begin by applying underwrap approximately 10 cm above and below your partner's elbow (*see* fig 11.10a).

• Place anchors over this mesh taping, surrounding the arm by two thirds only.

• Bend your partner's elbow by 10 degrees (unload it) and from the anchors attach stirrups crossing in the centre of the elbow hollow (cubital fossa) (*see* fig 11.10b).

• Use one or two layers of stirrup, depending on the size and strength of your partner.

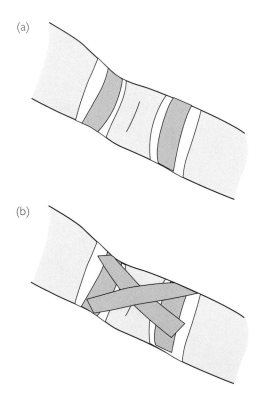

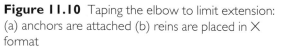

Figure 11.10 Taping the elbow to limit extension: (a) anchors are attached (b) reins are placed in X format

EXERCISES

Limited range arm curl

Purpose
To strengthen and shorten the arm flexor muscles.

Preparation
Begin holding a dumbbell in the hand of your affected arm.

Action
Bend (curl) your arm, attempting to touch your shoulder with the dumbbell (full inner range) (*see* fig 11.11a). Allow your arm to straighten but stop the movement short of full extension (20 degrees) by resting your exercising hand in your resting hand (*see* fig 11.11b). Perform 8–10 reps.

Tips
Perform the action slowly to maintain the exercise intensity on the muscle.

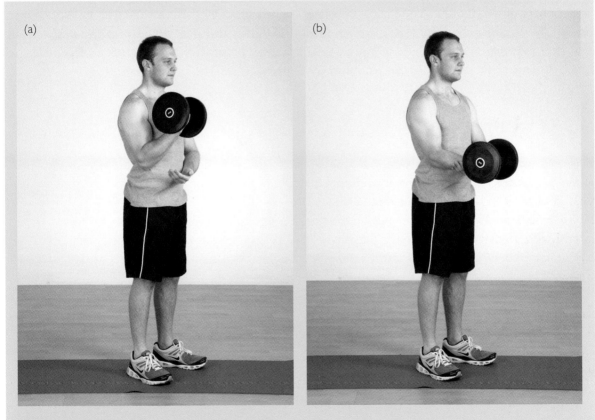

Figure 11.11 Limited range arm curl: (a) start position (b) mid position

NERVE CONDITIONS

There are three major nerves travelling within the forearm. On the thumb side is the *radial nerve*, on the little finger side is the *ulnar nerve*, and travelling down the centre of the forearm between the two is the *median nerve*. The nerves connect to a larger nerve coming from the neck, and travel into the hand for feeling (sensory) and movement (motor) of the fingers.

The radial nerve may be involved with tennis elbow pain and injury to the upper part of the radius bone, and gives pain into the thumb and first finger. Pain gets worse when the forearm is turned down (knuckles facing the ceiling) and the wrist is bent down (flexed). As we have discussed previously, the ulnar nerve travels in a small groove on the inner aspect of the elbow and can be involved with golfer's elbow, giving pain into the little finger. The median nerve is not commonly injured at the elbow, but commonly painful at the wrist (*see* chapter 12).

Pain may also occur from compression of the nerves in the neck after a whiplash injury or general neck pain. Although you feel pain in your forearm and often into your hand, the compression is higher up. Examination by a physiotherapist shows that your neck movements are unequal, with one side being stiffer to twist (rotation) and bend sideways (side bend), and sometimes you notice this in everyday actions such as reversing your car. Pain from trigger points around the back of the shoulder (rotator cuff) and upper spine may also give pain into the arm as far as the hand. These points may be found and relieved by massage into the local area.

Terms you should know:

Bursa – fluid-filled sac covering a body structure to avoid friction.

Hyperplasia – excessive healing, where tissue cells multiply more rapidly than expected following injury.

Pronation – twisting the forearm so the palm faces downwards.

Supination – twisting the forearm so the palm faces upwards.

Tinel's test – assessment of nerve irritation by light tapping (percussion) of the nerve. If positive, the subject feels a tingling sensation or 'pins and needles' along the course of the nerve. Commonly used over the median nerve at the wrist and ulnar nerve at the elbow.

WRIST AND HAND

12

The wrist consists of joints between the ends of the forearm bones (radius and ulna) and the block-like hand (carpal) bones, and between the individual carpal bones themselves (*see* fig 12.1). Each joint is strengthened by ligaments and controlled by muscles travelling from the forearm to the fingers. On the underside (palmar aspect) the carpal bones form a shallow curve which is covered by a fibrous band (flexor retinaculum). Together this structure is called the *carpal tunnel*, and through it run the long finger-bending tendons (flexors) and the median nerve. Compression of the nerve within the tunnel causes carpal tunnel syndrome as described below.

The main function of the fingers is to grip, and two categories of grip occur. *Precision grip* is applied using the tips, pads and nails of the fingers, working together as pincers. *Power grip* involves the whole hand: the wrist muscles work together to lock the wrist, and the fingers and thumb work together to pull the object into the centre of the palm.

A balance should exist between the finger-bending muscles (flexors) and finger-straightening muscles (extensors) so that the wrist stays straight as you grip. Often the extensor muscles are weaker than the flexors, causing the wrist to angle inwards,

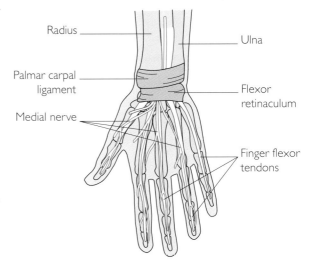

Figure 12.1 Structure of the wrist and hand

Keypoint

If the finger extensor muscles are weaker than the finger flexors, the wrist position during grip is altered. This change in wrist alignment is an important factor in painful repetitive wrist and forearm conditions.

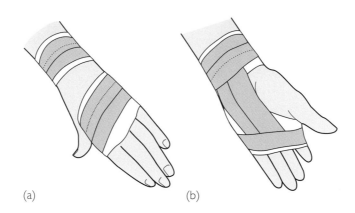

(a)   (b)

Figure 12.2 Wrist taping: (a) underwrap is used for protection while anchors are applied (b) taping should overlap stirrups

leaving you at risk of overuse conditions of the forearm and elbow.

WRIST SPRAIN

A wrist sprain may involve several structures, but most commonly it is an overstretching of the ligaments of the small block-like carpal bones (intercarpal ligaments). You feel pain when you bend (flex) your wrist, and there is often a tender spot between the bones at the root of the hand. Sometimes, if you fall onto your outstretched hand or press something forcefully, you can move one of the carpal bones out of place. This normally involves either the capitate or lunate bones in the centre of the wrist, and as the bones move they overstretch the ligaments holding them in place. You feel pain in the centre of your wrist in a line traced back into your wrist from your middle finger.

TAPING

Your wrist will only recover if it is rested in a supported position. When a carpal bone has

Keypoint

When a carpal bone has moved out of alignment you commonly feel pain in the centre of the back of your wrist on a line traced back from your middle finger.

moved out (subluxed) you will require a small manipulation from a physiotherapist to move it back in again. You will then need either a wrist taping or a commercial wrist brace which holds your wrist positioned slightly backwards (extended). The way to tape the wrist is to apply anchors around the wrist and hand with stirrups between the two (*see* fig 12.2).

- Begin by placing one piece of underwrap around your wrist just above the outer wrist knuckle (ulnar styloid) (*see* fig 12.2a).

- Place the second piece around your palm to the base of your thumb.

- Reinforce the underwrap with non-elastic tape placed two thirds around both your wrist and hand open on the underside (palmar aspect).

- Hold your wrist back slightly (20 degrees extension) and place two or three stirrups from hand to wrist, each overlapping the next by half of its width (*see* fig 12.2b, page 182).

- Finish the procedure by placing tape around your wrist and hand to cover the stirrup ends.

Your wrist should be held in slight extension, and you should find the tape stops you bending (flexing) your wrist more than 20–30 degrees. Keep the taping on for 3–5 days, and then allow the skin to recover before reapplying.

EXERCISES

The wrist needs to be strengthened for both extension and stability. Extension work involves fixing the forearm and moving the hand backwards, while stability uses the wrist locked while the arm is moving in several directions. Begin with wrist extensor strengthening (*see* page 173) and then progress to the wrist rolling exercise below.

Wrist rolling
Purpose
To strengthen the wrist extensor muscles and build endurance.

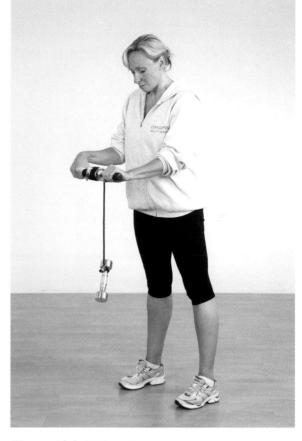

Figure 12.3 Wrist rolling

Preparation
Begin holding a wrist roller, with your elbows tucked into your sides, forearms horizontal and knuckles facing the ceiling.

Action
Wind the rope around the wrist roller by alternately bending and straightening (flexing and extending) your wrists (*see* fig 12.3). When the weight is at the top of the rope, reverse the action to gradually lower it to the ground.

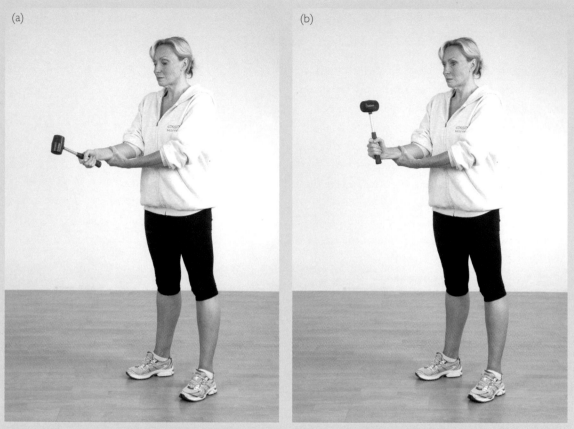

Figure 12.4 Hammer grip: (a) start position (b) mid position

Tips

If you allow your elbows to move, work is taken from the forearms to the upper arms.

Hammer grip

Purpose

To build stability in the wrist.

Preparation

Hold a hammer in your affected hand and keep your wrist locked (*see* fig 12.4a).

Action

Bend and straighten your elbow, with your knuckles facing in several directions (*see* fig 12.4b). Perform 15–20 reps, rest and then repeat.

Tips

Vary the speed of movement, performing some reps slowly and others more quickly to work on muscle reaction speed.

WRIST FRACTURE

The most common wrist fracture is that of the *scaphoid*, a block-like bone at the base of your thumb. If you look at the side of your hand (thumb on top) and pull your thumb upwards you will notice a hollow between the two thumb tendons (anatomical snuffbox). The scaphoid bone lies at the base of this hollow (*see* fig 12.5). The bone is fractured by falling onto your hand when it is fully pulled back into extension and locked, jamming the scaphoid between the thumb and the end of the outer forearm bone (radius). When the wrist is slightly movable, for example if you fall and slip, the end of the radius bone tends to fracture rather than the scaphoid. Although the scaphoid can be injured from a fall, it may also be injured by repeated forced extension such as occurs in a gymnastic vault, martial arts open hand strike or bench press in the gym.

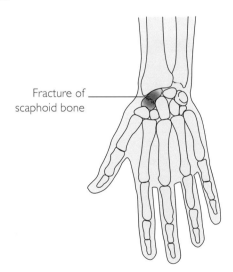

Fracture of scaphoid bone

Figure 12.5 Location of the scaphoid fracture

> **Keypoint**
>
> The most common fracture at the wrist is to the scaphoid bone at the base of the thumb.

Sometimes the fracture may be missed on a hospital X-ray as the line of the fracture can be very faint. When detected, the position of the break is important, because on occasions the blood flow to the bone may be damaged, making healing very slow. Where healing is delayed you may need an operation to put a metal pin into the bone to support it. Normally, however, you simply need a plaster cast which covers your forearm, wrist and thumb.

After the bone has healed, the wrist is very stiff and weak because it has been immobile for a long period. You will require intensive physiotherapy to improve movement and grip, and exercise therapy is key to your successful return to sport.

EXERCISES

Thumb range of motion
Purpose
To begin thumb movements following prolonged immobilisation.

Preparation
Place a cushion or folded towel on your lap, and rest the back of your affected hand and forearm on it.

Action
Try to touch the tip of your thumb to the tip of each finger in turn, then to the middle of each

finger, and finally to the base of each finger. Use a continuous motion and perform each cycle 5 times.

Tips
At first your thumb will be very stiff and you may have little movement. It is important to continue the exercise, however, as movement will increase the flow of blood and tissue fluids to the area.

Assisted wrist bend
Purpose
To begin wrist flexion and extension.

Preparation
Begin with your hand flat on a table top, your wrist at the table edge. Place your unaffected hand on top of your injured one, with the fingers of the top hand at the edge of your wrist.

Action
Keeping your hand flat on the table top, move your elbow down (wrist flexion) and then upwards (wrist extension). Begin with small (1–2 cm) movements and gradually increase this as pain allows. Perform 5 sets of 5 reps each.

Tips
If you are unable to flatten your hand onto the table top completely, hold it as close as you can. Over time the range of motion will improve to enable you to practise the full exercise.

Assisted wrist side bend
Purpose
To begin wrist abduction and adduction.

Preparation
Begin with your hand flat in the centre of a table top, forearm resting. Place your unaffected hand on top of your injured one, with the fingers of the top hand at the edge of your wrist.

Action
Keeping your hand flat on the table top, move your elbow side to side (wrist abduction and adduction), sweeping your elbow across the table. Begin with small (1–2 cm) movements and gradually increase as your pain allows. Perform 5 sets of 5 reps each.

Tips
It is common to find movement to one side better than that to the other.

Grip strength
Purpose
To rehabilitate grip strength.

Preparation
Grasp a soft tennis ball or piece of foam rubber in your affected hand.

Action
Grip the ball, squeezing with all of your fingers and thumb. Hold the tight position for 5 seconds and then release. Rest and then grip between the thumb and each fingertip individually. Rest and then repeat the full cycle 3 times.

Tips
Where your grip is very weak, just pressing your fingers into the ball is sufficient.

Pushing action

Purpose
To rehabilitate wrist compression.

Preparation
Begin placing a cushion or piece of foam rubber against a wall. Place the flat of your affected hand against the cushion.

Action
Press into the cushion using the heel of your hand. Hold the compression for 3–5 seconds and then release. Rest and then press into the cushion rapidly and release rapidly, performing 10 reps in a rhythmical pumping action. Repeat the whole exercise cycle twice.

Tips
This exercise is designed to reduce pain (desensitize) in the area and increase your confidence in your wrist. Your wrist may ache slightly, but should not be painful. Where pain occurs, stop and rest for 1 day before trying again.

NERVE CONDITIONS

Pain at the wrist may come from nerve involvement. A trapped nerve in the neck can cause pain to travel (refer) down through the arm and into the hand and fingers. Equally, injury to the nerve further down in the upper arm or elbow can also cause referral into the same region and the hand. However, two specific conditions within the wrist itself are caused by nerve compression: *carpal tunnel syndrome* and *cyclist's palsy*.

The *carpal tunnel* is formed by the block-like carpal bones which curve inwards forming an arch. Over the top of this arch, forming a roof, is a thick tough piece of flesh called the *flexor retinaculum* (*see* fig 12.1, page 181). The tunnel formed protects the flexor tendons going to the fingers, and the median nerve travelling down the centre of the forearm and into the hand. If the tunnel becomes restricted through swelling, tissue tightness or injury, the median nerve is compressed and you feel pain and tingling into the palm of your hand and into your thumb and first two fingers. Gripping for long periods and holding your wrist at a fixed angle makes the pain and tingling of carpal tunnel syndrome worse.

Treatment depends on the severity of your injury. Mild conditions may be treated with tablets to reduce swelling and by physiotherapy to stretch the tight muscles. Severe conditions may require an operation to release the tightness.

When the condition has healed, exercise is needed to gradually restore the movements of the hand. The assisted wrist bend exercise (*see* page 186) and pushing action exercise (*see* page 187) help to restore both movement and your pressing ability.

Cyclist's palsy is a compression of the ulnar nerve on the little finger side of the hand and occurs in long distance cyclists particularly. Pain and tingling are felt into the 4th (ring) and 5th (little) fingers. The nerve is stretched and compressed by the position of cycling where the wrist is pulled backwards (extension) and towards the little finger (ulnar deviation) (*see* fig 12.6, overleaf). It is essential to set up your bike for optimal alignment to avoid overstretching. If your seat is too high, for example, you will take more weight onto your hands, making the condition more likely. Visit a specialist cycle shop during a quiet period and take time to have this done. Reduce the forces on your hands by wearing cycling gloves with shock absorbing gel inserts in the palms, and put extra padding on your handlebars.

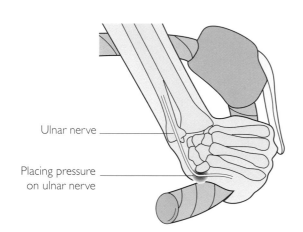

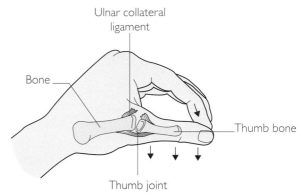

Ulnar nerve

Placing pressure
on ulnar nerve

Bone

Ulnar collateral
ligament

Thumb bone

Thumb joint

Figure 12.7 Thumb ligament injury

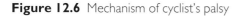

Figure 12.6 Mechanism of cyclist's palsy

THUMB PAIN

We have seen that fracture of the scaphoid bone at the base of the thumb can occur in sport. Injury to the thumb tendons is also common and is most often seen in skiing, hence the name *skier's thumb*. The injury occurs when the thumb is wrenched backwards away from the hand (abduction and extension) and typically occurs when you fall in skiing and your ski pole strap catches on your thumb. The ligament at the base of your thumb in the web space between your thumb and index finger (ulnar collateral ligament) is torn, leaving the lowest thumb joint unstable (*see* fig 12.7). You often notice that this joint moves excessively, giving a 'dip' in the joint as you grip something between your thumb and index finger (pinch grip), and your grip strength is substantially reduced. If the thumb is pulled back with less force, the ligament is sprained and not ruptured. In this case, the injury is called *gamekeeper's thumb* as it often used to occur as an overuse injury at the end of the season before protective splints and taping were used.

Less severe injuries may be managed using rest and protective taping. Complete rupture may require an operation. In both cases thumb exercise is needed afterwards to ensure that full grip strength returns.

TAPING

Thumb taping aims to protect the thumb from being pulled back, but still allow an unhindered grip. Two tapes may be used: *continuous* (*see* fig 12.8, page 189) and *strip* (*see* fig 12.9, page 189). Continuous tape to the thumb (a spica) is rapid to apply but less precise. It is the type used before a game which stays on for a few hours only.

- For continuous taping, begin using non-elastic tape around the wrist starting on the little finger side (ulna side).

- Take the tape around the back (dorsum) of the hand to the outside of the first thumb joint (1st MP joint).

- Bring the tape across the palm and then back to the little finger side of the wrist.

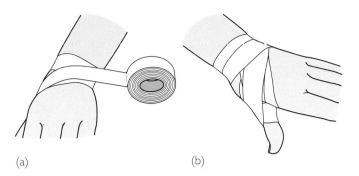

Figure 12.8 Continuous thumb taping: (a) non-elastic tape is placed around wrist (b) taping encircles the thumb

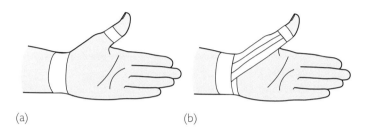

Figure 12.9 Strip taping: (a) the two anchors (b) overlapping reins join the anchors

- Perform two or three circuits of this tape, finishing with an anchor strip around the wrist.

Strip taping is more variable, enabling you to alter the tension of the tape on your partner's thumb. Varying the position of the strips enables you to more accurately dictate the thumb movement. For strip taping, place anchors around the wrist and the middle or end bone (phalanx) of the thumb (*see* fig 12.9a).

- Place three strips of tape from the wrist, across the palm to the thumb anchor.

- Finish by reinforcing the anchors with second pieces of tape (*see* fig 12.9b).

Following removal of the tape, the thumb must be re-strengthened. Exercises for general grip strength and finger-thumb (opposition) strength are practised. Thumb stability is also enhanced.

EXERCISES

Thumb stability press
Purpose
To enhance thumb stability and stop the thumb joints from giving way.

Preparation
Begin by placing a thick piece of foam or a cushion on a table top.

Action

Keep your injured thumb locked out straight, and press the end of the thumb into the foam. First press perpendicular to the foam and then at varying angles. Do not press so hard that the thumb joints bend.

Tips

Very gentle pressure is needed to begin, because pressing the bones of the thumb joint together (approximation) after injury can be painful. Only press hard enough to work the thumb, not so hard that it is painful.

Repeated actions using the thumb or gripping can cause the sheath surrounding two thumb tendons to inflame – a condition called *tenosynovitis* (or *de Quervain's syndrome*). You feel pain and sometimes grating as you move your thumb, with pain focused over the base of the thumb and thumb side of the wrist. Pain is often made worse when you take your thumb across your palm towards the base of your little finger. This movement stretches the affected thumb tendons (abductor pollicis longus and extensor pollicis brevis), which normally work to pull the thumb out and back. Treatment aims to rest the area to allow recovery. Commercially available thumb splints hold the wrist and thumb still, and should be worn for 10–14 days while working (*see* fig 12.10). During this time you will benefit from deep massage to the area to break up thickened swelling. As pain eases, thumb tendon stretching is used to restore full movement, which is often lost during injury.

Thumb tendon stretch

Purpose

To lengthen the thumb tendons after injury.

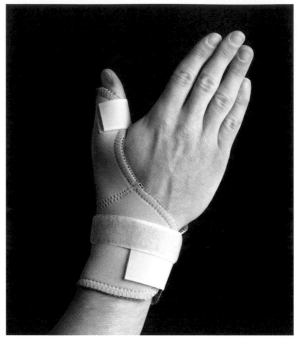

Figure 12.10 Thumb splint for tenosynovitis or thumb joint pain

Preparation

Begin resting your injured forearm on a bench, palm up.

Action

Take your thumb to the base of your little finger. Tip your wrist to the little finger side of your body (ulnar deviation). Put overload on the stretch by drawing both your thumb and your wrist further across, using your uninjured thumb at the inside of your wrist and uninjured fingers to draw your thumb across your palm (*see* fig 12.11, page 191). Hold the stretch for 20–30 seconds and then release. Perform 3 reps.

Tips

Combining this stretch with massage along the length of the tendon from above the wrist to the

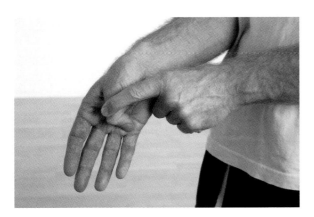

Figure 12.11 Thumb tendon stretch

- Begin by placing felt between the injured finger and the one next to it. The felt fills in the gaps between the knuckles and makes sure that the knuckle bones do not rub together. If you do not have felt, thick cotton wool will do.

- Place one piece of non-elastic tape around the bottom (proximal) finger bone, finishing the tape on the back of the finger.

- Place a second piece around the middle bone, again finishing on the back of the hand.

When the taping is in place, you should be able to gently bend your fingers but feel supported. If you feel throbbing in your fingers the tape is too tight and should be removed straight away.

thumb itself can help increase the range of motion and reduce pain.

FINGER JOINT DISLOCATION

Finger joints can often be 'put out' or dislocated in contact sports or if the tip of your finger is hit by a ball. Most commonly it is the little (5th) finger which is involved, and the finger is forced backwards (posterior dislocation). Usually the joint simply dislocates, but sometimes a small chip of bone may come away from the joint. For this reason, gentle traction (pulling) should be applied along the length of the finger. If it goes back (reduces) easily that is fine. However, if the finger does not go back straight away, you will need to go to hospital to have an X-ray to check that the bone is not chipped. Even if the finger has gone back it is important to get if checked by your doctor to ensure that the finger is not damaged.

TAPING

Taping is used to support the finger and allow it to recover, and the easiest to put on is *buddy taping* (*see* fig 12.13, page 193).

FINGER TENDON INJURY

Finger tendons may be injured, but forcing actions tend to dislocate the joint. However, tendon injury to the fingers is particularly rife in rock climbing, where the tendon 'pulleys' are involved. The long finger-bending (flexor) tendons intertwine together as they travel from the wrist and hand towards the fingertips. The tendons are held in place by tissue pulleys wrapping around the fingers (annular pulley) and crisscrossing the length of the finger (cruciform pulley). Each pulley is named with a letter to show which type it is: A1–A5 for annular and C1–C3 for cruciform. In rock climbing it is the A2 pulley (*see* fig 12.12a, overleaf) that is most commonly injured.

The A2 pulley is injured due to the type of grip used in rock climbing which is peculiar to this sport. The grip is called a *crimp* and involves holding onto a rock face just with the very tips of the fingers, which allows the end joint (distal inter-phalangeal

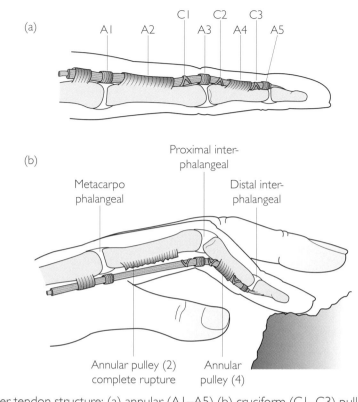

Figure 12.12 Finger tendon structure: (a) annular (A1–A5) (b) cruciform (C1–C3) pulleys

joint) to hyperextend or dip backwards, while the first finger joint (proximal inter-phalangeal joint) is flexed (*see* fig 12.12b). Once the injury has occurred rest is the first form of treatment, however, an operation may be required if the pulley has snapped rather than just strained.

TAPING

Taping is used to support your fingers, with the finger being held in flexion (bent) to avoid the hyperextension position that causes the damage.

- Using thin non-elastic tape, place a single stirrup around the pad of the end finger bone (distal phalanx).

- A length of tape (rein) is then placed beneath the finger and secured by a second stirrup around the first finger bone (proximal phalanx).

- The tape is held firm by a third stirrup around the middle finger bone.

Make sure that the stirrups avoid the joint creases so you can move your fingers unhindered. Also, the tape must not be put on so tightly that your finger circulation is reduced and you get throbbing in your fingers.

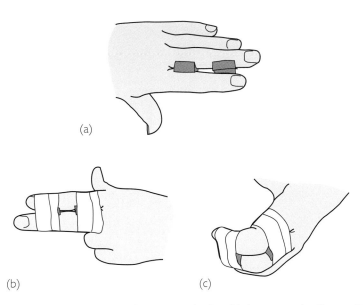

(a)

(b)   (c)

Figure 12.13 Buddy taping: (a) joint pressure is protected using felt between the fingers (b) tape strips avoid the knuckles (c) bending (flexion) movement is unhindered

Terms you should know:

Carpal tunnel – tunnel located at the wrist through which the flexor tendons and median nerve pass.

Crimp grip – grip used in rock climbing which stresses the fingertips.

Cyclist's palsy – compression of the ulnar nerve at the little finger side of the wrist.

de Quervain's syndrome (tenosynovitis) – (also called *washerwomen's wrist*) an inflammatory condition affecting the sheath around the major two thumb tendons.

Dislocation – bones in a joint becoming malaligned due to injury.

Finger pulley – specialised tissue holding finger tendons in place. There are two types: *annular* encircling the finger and *cruciform* crisscrossing the finger.

Interphalangeal joint – IP

Metacarpophalangeal joint – MP

Radial deviation – movement which pulls the wrist to the thumb side of the forearm.

Skier's thumb – tear of the ligament at the base of the thumb (ulnar collateral ligament)

Spica – taping or splint which immobilises a digit or limb together with the body part it attaches to. A thumb spica immobilises the wrist and thumb; a shoulder spica, the upper trunk and arm; and a hip spica, the lower trunk and leg.

Subluxation – bones in a joint becoming partially malaligned due to injury (also called *partial dislocation*).

Ulnar deviation – movement which pulls the wrist to the little finger side of the forearm.

// FURTHER INFORMATION

USEFUL READING

Bache TR and Earle RW (2008) *Essentials of Strength and Conditioning* (3rd edition). Human Kinetics. Champaign, Illinois.

Bean, A (2001) *The Complete Guide to Strength Training* (2nd edition) A&C Black Publishers, London.

de Domenico G, Woods EC (2004) *Beard's Massage* (4th edition). W.B. Saunders & Co. Ltd, London.

Levangie, PK and Norkin, CC (2011) *Joint Structure and Function*: *A comprehensive analysis* (5th edition). F. A. Davies, Philadelphia.

Norris, CM (2003) *Bodytoning: Principles and Practice.* A&C Black Publishers, London.

Norris, CM (2004) *Sports Injuries: Diagnosis and Management* (3rd edition). Butterworth Heinemann, Oxford.

Norris, CM (2007) *The Complete Guide to Stretching* (3rd edition). A&C Black Publishers, London.

Norris, CM (2009) *The Complete Guide to Abdominal Training* (3rd edition). A&C Black Publishers, London.

Norris, CM (2011) *Managing Sports Injuries.* Elsevier. Oxford.

Palastanga, N, Field, D, and Soames R (2006) *Anatomy and Human Movement* (5th edition). Elsevier, Oxford.

Peterson L, Renstrom P (2000) *Sports Injuries: Their prevention and treatment* (3rd edition). Martin Dunitz Ltd

Rolf, CG (2007) *The Sports Injuries Handbook: Diagnosis and Management.* A&C Black Publishers, London.

Tortora G (2003) *Principles of Human Anatomy* (8th edition). John Wiley and Sons, Oxford.

PRODUCT SUPPLIERS

Physio Supplies Ltd.
The Warehouse
Beck Bank
West Pinchbeck
Spalding
Lincolnshire, PE11 3QN
United Kingdom
Website: www.physiosupplies.com

Physio-Med Services Ltd
7-23 Glossop Brook
Business Park
Surrey Street
Glossop
Derbyshire, SK13 7AJ
United Kingdom
Website: www.physio-med.com

Physique Management Company Limited
Alexandria Park
Penner Road
Havant
Hampshire, PO9 1QY
United Kingdom
Website: www.physique.co.uk

Pro-Tec Athletics
Maverick Sports Medicine, Inc
dba Pro-Tec Athletics
18080 NE 68th St. #A150
Redmond, WA 98052
USA
Website: www.injurybegone.com

Swede-O, Inc
6459 Ash Street
North Branch
MN 55056, USA
Website: www.swedeo.com

Thumper Massager Inc.
BCL, 2 Las Palomas
Albert Rd
Bracknell, RG42 2AE
United Kingdom
Website: www.thumpermassager.com

USEFUL ORGANISATIONS

Chartered Society of Physiotherapy
14 Bedford Row
London, WC1R 4ED
United Kingdom
Website: www.csp.org.uk

Federation of Holistic Therapists
18 Shakespeare Business Centre
Hathaway Close
Eastleigh
Hampshire, SO50 4SR
United Kingdom
Website: www.fht.org.uk

Norris Associates
16 Lawton Street
Congleton
Cheshire, CW12 1RP
United Kingdom
Website: www.norrisassociates.co.uk

Sports Massage Association
1 Woodville Terrace
Lytham
Lancashire, FY8 5QB
United Kingdom
Website: www.sportsmassageassociation.org

INDEX OF EXERCISES

GENERAL INDEX

EPPING FOREST COLLEGE LIBRARY
BORDERS LANE, LOUGHTON
ESSEX IG10 3SA
Tel: 020 8508 8311

757365